"SHE DOESN'T SING ANYMORE"

"SHE DOESN'T SING ANYMORE"

◆

A Daughter's Journey with Her Mother Who Has Alzheimer's

Ernestine Williams-Burtley

iUniverse, Inc.

New York Lincoln Shanghai

"SHE DOESN'T SING ANYMORE"
A Daughter's Journey with Her Mother Who Has Alzheimer's

iUniverse books may be ordered through booksellers or by contacting:

iUniverse
2021 Pine Lake Road, Suite 100
Lincoln, NE 68512
www.iuniverse.com
1-800-Authors (1-800-288-4677)

Because of the dynamic nature of the Internet, any Web addresses or links contained in this book may have changed since publication and may no longer be valid.

The information, ideas, and suggestions in this book are not intended as a substitute for professional medical advice. Before following any suggestions contained in this book, you should consult your personal physician. Neither the author nor the publisher shall be liable or responsible for any loss or damage allegedly arising as a consequence of your use or application of any information or suggestions in this book.

ISBN: 978-0-595-44406-9 (pbk)
ISBN: 978-0-595-88736-1 (ebk)

Printed in the United States of America

To My Dad,
My sons, Harvey and David,
My daughter Hope and her husband, Doug
Thank you for your Love

"An Unknown Thief Robs Again
Stealing what they want.
Sometimes of value to them, sometimes not;
They hit in broad daylight
Most times in the dark."

By E. Williams-Burtley

Contents

FOREWORD

Accompanying someone with Alzheimer's disease can be compared to walking an unchartered path through an unknown forest. Ernestine Burtley writes a very personal, poignant memoir of her journey with her mother down this path full of sudden turns, and dead ends. She convinced me that it was a journey she could not have made without her faith in God. As I read, I kept picturing her holding onto her mother with her right hand, and the Lord holding onto her left hand. This is a must read for anyone caring for a person with Alzheimer's disease.

Chaplain Diane Jorgensen, BCC,MA,LMHP
Director of Spiritual Care and Coordinator of Psychiatric Services
Maple Crest Care Center
Omaha, Nebraska

ACKNOWLEDGEMENTS

I needed to be motivated beyond my comfort zone
I wish to thank these people for being that tool

My sister, Elizabeth McClodden
My Cousin, Art Andrews

And a special thanks to a special friend in Detroit
Who brought lost love back into my life.

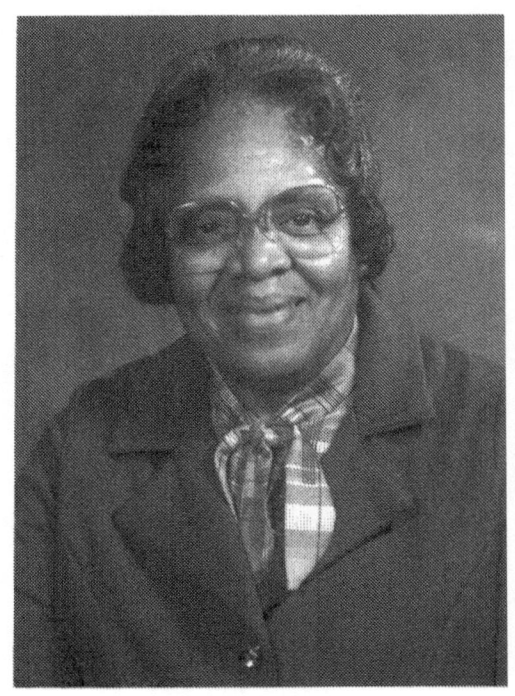

Eula Mae Williams (Samuel)

INTRODUCTION

It was the spring of 1996; I was sleeping lightly, resting for the next day's task and fighting thoughts of a relationship I need not be involved, silence surrounds my thoughts as I drift off to sleep. As the phone rings, hundreds of thoughts began to flood my mind within seconds. Believing that my children were all well and where they were supposed to be, I picked up the phone. On the other end was the voice of a distressed woman saying "Teen, can you come and get me please, come and get me." It was my mom. Only one other time had I heard such distress in her voice when she and Dad were having some marital problems some years ago. As I tried to calm and comfort her, I asked what was wrong and her reply was as always, she missed us. It was then I realized that there is something changing in her life. I had never felt this helpless before. My first instinct was to jump into my car and go, but traveling 1,100 miles by car was out of the question and airline tickets at such short notice was not within my price range. I didn't want to tell her I couldn't come right then. I tried to comfort her to the best of my ability talking more on other subjects like the grandchildren. Our conversation ended with prayer and telling her I would be home in a few weeks which seemed to satisfy her. *"Love you mom and stay prayerful."*

It had only been a few years that she and dad had moved back to Alabama after living in Omaha for more than 37 years; and it was only a few months before mom's condition was to be diagnosed as probable Alzheimer's disease.

Inspired to Write

My purpose in writing is threefold. First and foremost it is for my personal healing. During the time of caring for my mother, the only release I found was in writing down what was happening to her, to me and the rest of the family on a daily basis. In sharing this book with others, is in no way disrespect to my mom or my family but it is to let others know of my encounter of caring for a loved one with Alzheimer's disease. I have gained much understanding and comfort in the books I have read, but none of them tell my story. Some things which happened should not be mentioned or even written on paper. But it is my hope that knowing in advance or having some idea of what to expect, perhaps my writing will help you in your decision should this lot ever fall upon you.

Secondly, to speak out and share with others, who find themselves as caregivers, the fact that it can be done. No longer be silent or ashamed when a loved one is living with Alzheimer's disease. Yes we have the faith to believe that God can heal all types of disease, but should it not be in his perfect plan, how do we deal with and/or live with this disease which has affected so many of our loved ones. Although sometimes it may seem a lonesome task, you are not alone and the ability to ask for help is one step in the right direction. When dealing with a loved one with Alzheimer's disease, you will experience a whole range of emotions, including anger, frustration, impatience, embarrassment and avoidance. It will definitely require a personal commitment. Dr. Martin Luther King Jr. said "**the ultimate measure of man is not where he stands in moments of comfort and convenience, but where he stands at times of challenge and controversy**."

Third, in sharing with my children and relatives about a lady we all know and love, gives them information to pass on to their children. I want to leave behind some family medical background for future reference. Also, I want them to know that while my mother is slowly declining, there is still life and she deserves the best I can give. She needs my time and assistance in remembering all those special notable moments in her life. It is the past and the hope of the future that keeps us going—I can still hear my mother's voice some years ago, when she awakening from a deep sleep, told me "I'm back, I am ready to take control of my life again"—"*I awoke and behold it was a dream*" (*John Bunyan*).

Alzheimer's disease has all the traits of a thief with a unique strategy which is planned long before the attack. And like any thief, they don't weigh the consequences; but eventually will be caught. This thief stole the song from singing lips, the praise from clapping hands and dancing feet, he then stole my mom. How many attacks will be made before he is captured?

1

A WOMAN YOU SHOULD KNOW

o o o o o o o o o o o o o o o o o o o o o o o o o o o o o o o o o o

"My lips shall greatly rejoice when I sing unto thee; and my soul, which thou hast redeemed. My tongue also shall talk of thy righteousness all the day long ..."

—*Psalms 71:23–24*

Where do I start has always been an issue with me. If I start too far back then my memory lapses and if I start at the present, then you won't know the person I am writing about. Of all the challenges in life, writing of a life's experience has not been top of my list until now and this is something I must do. I want to share with you my experiences with a lady whom I have loved since birth. She is known by many names: Mrs. Eula Mae Williams, Sister Williams, Missionary Williams, Aunt Babe, Baby, or Eula. For me, it has always been "Mama." She is my queen, my role model and my teacher. She was born on December 26, 1929, in Conecuh County, Alabama, the fourth child born to Clinton and Mary Lee Samuel and the granddaughter of Washington and Emma Samuel.

In order to know my mom you have to know the man she married and loved until now. She and my dad were married in November of 1948 and were blessed with three children. My dad, Arnold Williams Jr. left school while in the 9th grade which was quite common then—the boys of larger families worked during the planting and harvesting seasons to help their family. His family lived south of Evergreen, Alabama in the rural area called the Franklin Town Settlement. It was told me that my grandfather, Papa Arnold as he is called, was one of the first Negro business men in the area. He bought a school bus and contracted with Conecuh County to drive the colored children to school. When my dad became

1

of age, he began driving the bus in which my mom rode and this was the beginning of the courtship between him and my mom.

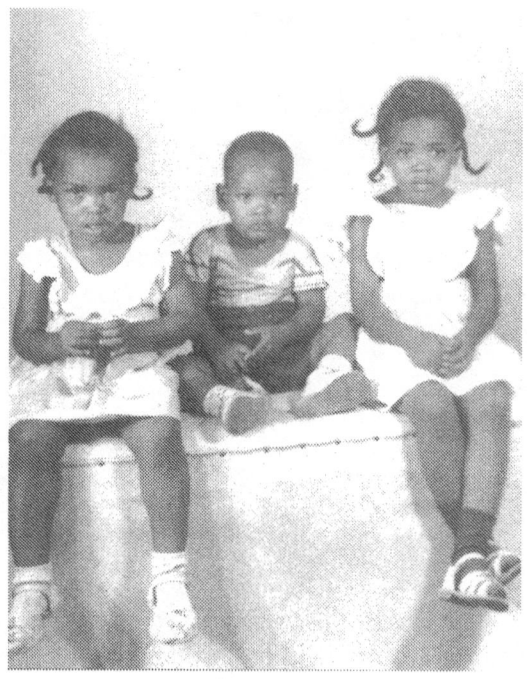

"Her Babies" (1954)

My father like most men in that area was a strong man, both physically and mentally. He was taught to take care of his family no matter what, which he did very well. In the early 1950's being a strong willed black man in the Deep South sometimes brought trouble, leaving him with a desire to leave. It was through some distant cousins that my dad received word that there were jobs up north. Many family members had already moved to Cincinnati, Detroit and Omaha. He left the Johnsonville community in early summer 1955 coming to Omaha, Nebraska to later send for his wife and children.

Growing up, I remember Mom as a great cook, always trying something new. If there was a food she didn't eat, we didn't have it at our house with the exception of turnip greens and okra. She didn't eat the turnip greens but loved the roots; and okra was totally out but she prepare theses dishes for the family because one, it was one of dad's favorites and it made good wholesome meals. She loved the "Family Circle" magazine with all of their great recipes and home ideas.

Any recipe that caught her eye, she would try it on her family. Many of her favorite foods she passed on to me, especially sweet potatoes, peanuts and pecans. My grandfather knew she loved white sweet potatoes and wouldn't start digging them up until "Baby comes home." As I was told, she didn't much like working in the fields picking cotton as the others but spent a lot of time in the kitchen helping prepare meals and other family chores. Perhaps that's why she is such a good cook.

The Singer and Composer

There have been many times that I wish that I had listened more carefully and attentive to her words as I was growing up, letting her words of wisdom saturate and linger until now. Having to spend as much time with Mom now, makes me realize how much I do not know about her. What were her feelings on certain issues about life, her relationship with our dad or even what her thoughts were on politics? But one thing I do know, she loved to sing. It was who she was. You could always find her singing a solo, in a group or a choir—singing first and sometimes second soprano.

When I was a little girl around the age of four or five, there was a group of ladies who would come to our home in the back woods of Johnsonville (which still stands today abandoned) on a regular basis. While we were out running around doing what toddlers do, they would be on the porch singing many gospel songs of old.

Most of our family members attended the Sandy Grove Baptist Church. In fact when she and dad were married, she was singing in the choir there. When we relocated to Omaha, she joined the Faith Temple Church of God in Christ choir, doing what she loved to do.

Over the years she had written many gospel songs which were a witness of the life we all should live. Once, during one of my visits to Alabama, I asked what happened to all the songs that she had written. Knowing exactly where they were, she went into her room and brought them out with joy and excitement. She carefully spread them out on the table pointing out a few. I was familiar with some of them and others I asked her to sing a course or two. Each one I picked up, she'd sing the songs she was inspired to write, knowing the tunes in which she had composed for each one. Mom had never taken music lessons, but she was blessed with the ability to write and sing songs. Two of her songs were published and recorded with the first one entitled "Jesus Is Coming Again" *(Don Sears Record-*

ing, Omaha, Nebraska, 1968) and a few years later the second one was entitled "Sanctify Me Lord" *(Savoy Record Company)*. This is my favorite:

Song: Jesus is Coming Again!

Chorus:
Have you heard about Jesus, (Jesus is coming Again) (3X)
He is coming on a cloud every eye shall see Him
Glory Hallelujah, He's coming again, so soon.
Verse 1:
Listen let me tell you, just what the bible says,
He's coming on cloud every eye shall see him
Glory Hallelujah, he's coming again so soon.
Repeat Chorus:
Verse 2:
Listen, let me tell you, just what the bible says,
He's coming as a thief and robber by night, the hour we know not when.
Repeat Chorus:
Special:
Jesus (He's coming) He's Coming (He's coming)
Be ready (He's coming) He's Coming (He's coming)
Be faithful (He's coming) He's Coming (He's coming)
Be prayerful (He's coming) He's Coming (He's coming)
Be ready (He's coming) He's Coming (He's coming)
He is coming on a cloud every eye shall see Him
Glory Hallelujah, He's coming again, so soon.

Written by Eula Williams

Her Many Other Attributes of Womanhood

Mom always carried herself as a lady. Unlike me, she loved bright colors, lots of red, purples and greens—she wore quite a bit of plaid and flower patterns. I have always known her to be a healthy woman with big hips and great legs. In the earlier days you would sometimes find her in hats which complimented her round face and peach colored skin with cheek bones that reached her eyes. Her smile was enough to make anyone respond with a smile.

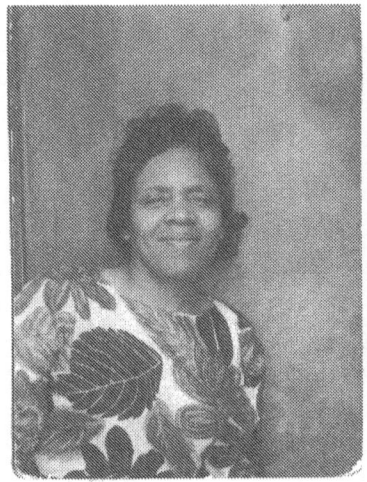 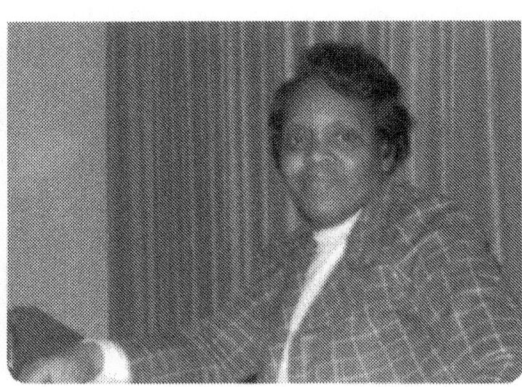

A young woman in the mid 1960's

Although singing was her love and favorite pastime, she worked in the house-keeping departments of Methodist Hospital and the downtown Fontenelle Hotel. As she became more familiar with the big city, she obtained several personal clients who all respected her for her honesty and commitment to her job. Day after day she made her way to her job which at times took her a far distance from home. Her last employer of more than twenty years (John & Betty Kaplan), remained in contact with her after she and dad moved back to Alabama.

Mom also was blessed with the talent of sewing. There was always an operative sewing machine in our house. She felt that every woman should have the ability to sew and made sure my sister and I knew how; helping us with our homemaking projects with ease. Her favorite time to sew was late at night, but its funny I never remember any noise at night … she was very quiet. I guess it was less distractions during those late hours. I remember my sister and I would always have two dresses for Easter, one for the morning service and the other for the Easter program which at that time was always that Sunday afternoon. She would purchase one from the department store and make the other. She had a tendency to dress Sister and myself alike, and being only a year apart, people thought we were twins.

Religion. Mom had accepted Christ into her life after she and dad were married. Often she would mention the traveling evangelist by the name of Elder Pleasant, and how he came through the area conducting a revival in which she accepted Christ as her savior. After relocation to Omaha, she joined the Faith Temple Church of God in Christ, under the leadership of Elder Vernon Richardson. People knew that church was her life in the way she lived. She loved the church, what it represented and the opportunities it afforded her in expressing her many talents. Besides being a singer and composer, she had great clerical skills and was very good in math which qualified her to hold the position of church secretary for many years. Whenever the doors opened at the church, she was there and somehow she still managed to visit the sick, help clean someone's house, visit relatives and had time to talk and laugh with her friends—we never went lacking of her care and attention.

Her faith in God was shared many times in her songs and personal testimony; praising God in a way that one knew she was appreciative of God's love. There were some periods in her life during the early 70s which seemed to be hard and sometimes unbearable for her. Many times crying when she could not go to church but she remained faithful to God and submissive to her husband, which always take you to another level in your faith walk. I remember her witnessing to someone how that she physically went on the back porch, looked up to heaven and asked God "Are you coming soon" which possibly inspired the lyrics to the song, "Jesus Is Coming Again." She studied God's word faithfully and her prayer life was that of a woman who knew the power of prayer. She was also a fasting woman who realized that the inner man needs to be brought to the forefront.

As an evangelist missionary in the church, she presented the word of God with authority and tried to live by precept and example. When she did give advice, she'd refer to the Bible, and given the right subject she would give her own personal opinion. She was very liberated in her thoughts; saying things like "do it as unto the Lord" or "that's between you, your husband and God." In going through my own personal issues with divorce, her advice was limited being the Christian woman she was. She did not advise me much on my decision for a number of reasons, one was she knew first hand of my relationship and also, with her experiencing similar issues in her own life. But her words to me would always be "be encouraged, hold on to God and pray."

Shopper. Mom knew how to "bargain buy" and if she couldn't afford something to wear or put it on layaway, she would make it. The mail order catalogs were her friends because she stayed in-debt to "Fingerhut" and J.C. Penney. We all remember Fingerhut, order one thing and you are on their mailing list forever. The catch was "sign here and make small payments forever". But she always paid her bills. I sometimes wonder how she bought all the things that she did on such a small income. One reason was that she believed in paying her tithes, little or much or even playing catch-up, she was faithful. She learned early paying your tithes (1/10th of your earnings) was an act of your faith and believed in the power of being obedient to the Word of God, however way it was presented.

Education. Completing only the eleventh grade, she returned to school at the age of fifty-eight and obtained her GED in August 1988. With all she was involved, late evenings you would find her doing her math and English assignments. She spoke, read and wrote fluently and was very good in math. After graduation, she enrolled at the local community college and completed a couple of seamstress classes.

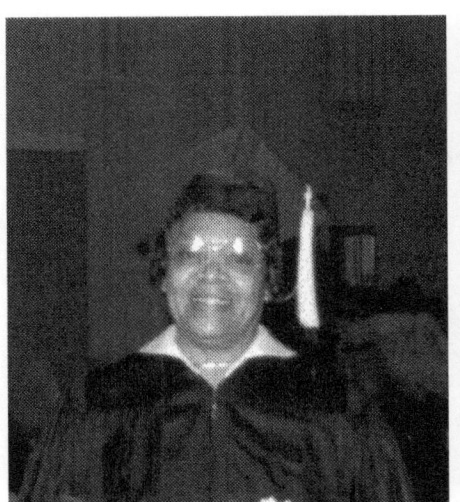 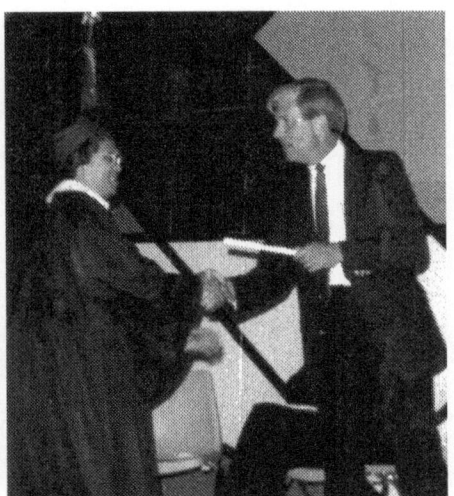

Graduation Day, her proud moment of achievement

My Mother and Friend

I always knew that mom was in my corner and would be there for me whenever I needed her. I can remember times when I'd need to get away from my husband and kids for whatever reason—I would go to mom and dad's house, go directly down into the sitting room, get on her soft sofa she had refurbished, wrap up in her sofa blanket and go to sleep. She seldom said anything or asked any questions, just continued what she was doing. But there were times she would follow me downstairs to sit and watch television with me, feeding me with her presence and praying for me. But now the lady I knew as a mother and friend, the woman who said "you need to pray about it" is slowly drifting away and life is reversing the role of mother and friend.

2

BEGINNING DOWN AN UNKNOWN PATH

o o o o o o o o o o o o o o o o o o o o o o o o o o o o o o o o o o o o

"With every beginning there is an end, but what matters most is what is within."

Mom's journey began long before we ever became aware of her having problems with her memory and long before she was diagnosed with Alzheimer's disease.

Moving Back to Alabama

After living in Omaha, Nebraska for more than thirty seven years, Dad and Mom moved back to the state of Alabama in May of 1992. This was always a dream of my father to relocate after he retired but he waited until mom reached age sixty two. It appeared she was adjusting well and when I call her response was always "I'm staying busy around the house, taking care of Hick" who she thought was working himself to death and "Aunt Hattie" who was very ill. It was later that we learned of my mother's unhappiness in moving back.

She would drive 10–15 miles in the morning to cook breakfast for Aunt Hattie and Uncle Lois, wash their clothes and hang them out on the line to dry. Then prepare lunch for both of them, pick up a little and about 2:00 PM was heading back up to town. After a few years passed, we could tell that it was taking a toll on her and began to really notice the changes in her behavior. It was then my sister and I convinced her to stop or at lease reduce the days to maybe once or twice a week. After other arrangements were made for Aunt Hattie's care, she was no longer needed but she continued to visit on a regular basis.

I have such fond memories of my visits to their home in Evergreen, how she would drive me around, knowing all the directions to go, showing no fear ... heading for the Kmart and the Wal-Mart stores located in Brewton. She would even drive the sometimes scary road to her sister Carrie's house, where there are no street lights on the rural routes and driving at night required some expertise. If you made a wrong turn, you could be lost for hours.

Early Detections

Getting Lost. There was one particular incident in Evergreen, where mom got confused while driving and couldn't find her way home. In one of our later conversations, she said that she started praying and asking God to show her where she was. God met her at her point of need and came to her rescue by helping her to remember where she was.

There was another time when her car stopped out on the road, and she got a ride back into town with some stranger. This really scared Dad, so he started taking her down to Aunt Hattie's each day to work and picked her up when she was done.

Mom would drive the distance to church or where ever she had to go, most times alone. The only way to keep her from driving was that the car was not running. One day, Dad had unhooked something underneath the hood and stalled getting it fixed. When I first heard of this, I thought it was so cruel of him to do that and resented him for the actions he took. I did not know what really had led up to this decision but I later realized the strain my dad was under and I thanked him for caring enough for her safety. Perhaps there was other ways that this could have been handled, but being new at this, it was the best solution at the time.

Money Matters. During the summer of 1995, she had begun having problems balancing her checking account. Once again, I should have known that something major was wrong because that was one area that she had no problems in the past. As it was, she would have the money but the deposits were always made late or she'd write checks and not log it in her checkbook, so when the overdrafts started coming, she didn't know how to handle it. I tried to keep her account balanced by sending money directly to her account. I closed this account on October 20, 1995.

I often wondered why Mom wouldn't let Dad help her and she began trusting him less, not that he was dishonest in any way. He is the most honest, fair man I know in this world. This is one of the symptoms of Alzheimer's disease, they feel something is being taken away from them. Dad would just give her just enough for pocket change which was a good idea because she would have given everything in her purse. She would go to the store and purchase items, and give large bills (10s or 20s) because she no longer could count out the correct amount.

Return Visits to Omaha. After relocating to Alabama, there were many return visits to Omaha, as frequently as twice a year. I'd send her an airline ticket and off she'd come. During those visits, I would plan her days to include visits with friends and leave things for her to do during the day. Each day I would come home and have lunch with her—She would be sitting in the swing on the porch waiting for me to arrive. As years past, arrangements would have to be made for part of the day. In the afternoon I'd take her over to a friend until I got off work so she would not have to be alone all day. I tried not to let her know I was afraid of leaving her alone. She would venture out to walk down the street to the home of a family friend, Dorothy Williams or she would go next door to Mrs. Morgan, who would do mom's hair, sit and chat a while then she'd return to the house.

The following summer and remaining times I would ask her about coming, she would start giving excuses and finally said she didn't want to come by herself. That is when my aunt Annie Lois became her travel companion. This was also an indication that things were not the same.

The Wedding Dress. It was the spring of 1995 and Mom flew to Omaha early to help in the preparation for my daughter's wedding … we had a wonderful time making the preparations. Yes she was having problems remembering, but times were good. Back in December, I had sent her some very expensive material and pattern, to make her dress for the wedding. She had assured me that she would have it completed before she came out here the first of March. Over the course of the next few months, I'd call and ask how she was coming. Her responses started out "will start on it soon" and then "it's all cut out." Early in January, when I called I asked how the dress was coming and she still had not completed the dress. In February during one of our conversations, she said she was working on it.

When Mom arrived at the airport, we returned to the house and helped her get settled in. It was after I saw what was done to the dress that I knew something was terribly wrong. The pattern pieces had been cut wrong and most of it had not been sewed. I could tell by the expressions on her face, how disappointed she was that she could not finish the dress. Being a professional seamstress, she never had problems sewing, especially something like this. There had been times when she would take a pattern and even rearrange it to fit her size and taste in fashion. I relieved some of her tension by telling her we would finish the dress together. I tried to sort the pattern out, but some of the pieces were missing. After awhile I told her we were going shopping for a dress and that pleased her so much. We found her a beautiful off white dress and hat that suited her fine. She was absolutely stunning at the wedding, and my dad was handsome as ever.

August 1997

There was one particular summer night I called Mom and asked her to read a few scriptures and to pray with me. She always had a joy in reading God's word and did it so eloquently, putting emphasis in the right places. When she finished reading, I asked her to lead us in prayer. Being the woman of faith that she is, she knew how to pray. After the prayer was ended and we were ready to say goodbye, she said "thank you dear, for all you do for me." As the tears began to run down my cheeks, there is comfort in knowing that she is aware of these little things we do.

The Big Meeting (October 15, 1997)

It is because of the fond memories I have of the "Big Meeting," that I made a special trip home to Evergreen, Alabama. This time of year, families from all over came back home for the big revival. Whenever I return to Sandy Grove Baptist Church, I just let my mind go back and imagine looking over to the left where you would see the front rows lined with these "great men of character" many of which were my great uncles. Three of these men stood out grand and tall; my grandfathers Papa (Arnold Williams) and Granddad (Clinton Samuel); then there was my Uncle (Lois Williams) who stood the tallest. Glancing over to the right, the entire front rows were filled with the "women of courage," my Grandmothers Lizzie Williams and Mary Lee Samuel. But the queen for a lifetime was Aunt Hattie Mae Williams. This church was larger than usual since it had so many families from the community like the Samuels, Williams', Jones', Likely family, and can't forget the Bradleys, just to mention a few.

Another reason for coming back at this time was to check on Dad and Mom. I did find both of them doing well, having all their ills under control. Dad was exceptionally glad to see me. As he embraced me, he held me so tight as if he didn't want to let go; maybe he did it all the time and I was just more aware of it now. I could see how Mom is slowly changing, a little more quiet than usual. She also was glad to see me but not her usual outgoing self.

I could tell that she wasn't taking a bath on a regular basis and that was a concern. My aunt, Annie Lois would come over now and then helping out when dad and mom would let her. She needed direction or she won't complete certain task. It took some additional time to help her, even to the point of running her bath water, setting her clothes out and helping her dress. She has always been very concerned about and very conscience of her appearances, personal care and hygiene. The first time I offered to help her in this way was a year ago when she came to Omaha. Seeing her nakedness, I found myself feeling embarrassed, but then I thought to myself this is my mom and she needs my help.

Even during this trip, she wanted so much to look her best and was constantly asking me "is this okay, does this look right?" I believe she changed clothes three or four times a day. Clothes would be left on the bed because making a decision on what to wear was becoming more difficult. Surprisingly, after all that she would put on the same thing she had on the day before.

Wednesday was quickly approaching and Mom knew it was getting close to time for me to go. As we were sitting around, she told me that she is going to miss me very much. It was said with so much emphasis that it really caused me concern. Could it be that she was lonely just sitting at home day and night with nothing to do and getting frustrated at task she is not able to complete. Dad was not much company. He could watch sports on television all day long as she just wonders around, when in the past she was always occupying her time with a hobby, visiting and going to church. Here is a woman who was accustomed to getting in her own car and going where she wanted; whether it was going to the Crossroads to shop, South Omaha to attend church services or the drive to work at Lake Manawa, it mattered not, she was on the go.

As we were sitting at the table talking over a light snack which included one of her favorite fruit, an apple. I gave her the knife to slice her apple as she has always traditionally done. Because of her upper partial smaller slices were easier to bite. Dad asked me to peel it for her which was no problem, but I wondered why. Then she looks at me and mumbles, "He acts like I can't do anything." I gave her the knife and she peeled the apple just find. The last evening of my visit was spent at church.

Christmas Celebration

Growing up, holidays at our house was always a big celebration with lots of family and friends. Christmas was one of the most festive of all the seasons of the year. It was time for shopping, decorating and cooking. Decorating the house was always enjoyable for Mom; what really brought her most joy was not only family, but the friends of family getting together, laughing, playing games and eating.

Mom was always using her creative ideas to prepare some new and traditional dishes to share with who ever came by. I remember the time she introduced her "miracle garden salad" using miracle whip, frozen peas, grated cheese, green onions and bacon bits with lots of lettuce. From then on, everyone looked for that dish first on the menu. An important thing to remember about Mom is that she believed in preparation. She would start up to thirty days in advance, preparing her menu and shopping for all the necessary ingredients.

Her fruitcakes were the "bomb" and no one could measure up to hers. It is hard to get children to eat fruit cake and even adults, but hers were eaten by everyone. After she had baked the cakes, there were times she had resorted to hiding the cakes in different locations, because they were eaten so fast. When the holiday celebrations began, we thought the cakes were all eaten up but at Christmas, a fruit cake always appeared. Her secret was to make lots of samplers. She would make sure a fruit cake was mailed to us in time to store them for a few days, if there was any left. Even when my eldest son was stationed in South Korea, she made sure that a fruitcake and cookies reached him at Christmas. Those cakes kept coming even after she and dad had moved back to Alabama.

Holiday Plans (December 1, 1997)

Earlier this year, I thought it would be a great idea to spend Christmas with my sister Liz in Los Angeles, California. She had been there quite some years, spending many of her holidays away from family. As the year progressed, I included mom and dad who were living in Alabama and my niece Kendra who had never been to California. I love to share first time experiences with people I love.

Disappointment (December 15, 1997)

It seems the closer it came time to go to California, the more difficult situations got. I purposely called Dad about ten days prior to leaving to make sure they didn't need anything. I could pick up these last minute items here before we departed. Mom & Dad were to fly to Omaha and then we all would travel together to California for Christmas. Then the breaking news came, Dad said that he could not make the trip with mom, he just could not handle it. I'm thinking what's to handle since I had arranged everything—go to Montgomery, get on the plane and come, what's hard about that? Those were my selfish thoughts. I found myself in a dilemma; the tickets are paid for and non-refundable—so what if we lose a few hundred dollars. Also, Kendra was going, and to cancel the trip would be disappointing to her. I then asked Dad to just to fly here with her and he can stay a few days and return home. The fact that Dad backed out caused me some worry about how Mom was going to get to Omaha. I desperately wanted her to go even if he didn't. It was only when I decided to let God work it out, that things came together.

Thank God for a willing son. David, who heard of my dilemma and agreed to fly down and pick mom up. I bought him a round trip ticket and off he went. Even with the additional cost of his ticket was less than what I'd loose if they didn't go. In the past, on occasions David, as a little boy had traveled with mom on the bus to Alabama. This time was no different except he was now grown and she has Alzheimer's disease. He loves his "Granny" as she is called. After he left, I called my Aunt Annie Lois to ask her to help mom pack. It was later that I learned that after mom was all packed, they were ready to go to the Montgomery airport and couldn't find one of her luggage and had to leave it. Dad returning home from the airport, found it hidden behind the sofa. I had wondered why she had come all this way with no under garments. She had really begun hiding things a lot.

I was doing all I knew to make it easy for them and I felt that Dad had let me down again. Actually what it was, my plans were not being followed through. I had no idea of what pressures my dad was under at that time and later I thank him for enduring as long as he did. Once again I see how selfish and ignorant my thoughts and actions were. The old saying goes and it holds true today, *"You never know the road one has traveled until you have travel that same road."*

David and Mom returned to Omaha within a couple of days. It was so funny, David was living about three hours away in Kearney, Nebraska at the time, so when they arrived at the airport, he didn't stop—he dropped her off and kept going. It is hard for a young person to understand Alzheimer's disease when they have known these individuals all their lives. He later told us of his return trip with "Granny." While waiting at the airport in Atlanta, Granny kept asking the same questions over and over. Where are we going? Where is Hick (nickname for my dad)? She told him she was leaving and in his frustrations, he told her to go ahead. He watched her as she walked away not letting her out of his sight. After awhile she came back and sat down with him until they departed.

Mom, Kendra and I left for Los Angeles, to have a good time with my sister, Liz for Christmas. Mom was getting more repetitive in her questions, wondering where Hick was. The flight was good and without incident. Kendra now sixteen years old, helped with mom a great deal. She was always close to mom and dad, being the youngest grandchild.

It is always amazing to fly into LAX, coming in over the ocean seeing everything so green and beautiful. Seems like a different world with all the hustle and bustle, which is totally different from the Midwest, where we can get anywhere within the city limit in thirty minutes.

We found Liz doing well and excited to see us. Mom was glad to see her also, but still quite puzzled about being here ... and yes, she recognized her other daughter. Liz had purchased a new home which I had not yet seen. When we saw it, oh my, what a beautiful home it is. She saw the potential of this place and God made it a reality. I am so proud of her and her accomplishments. The house is all decorated with Christmas lights everywhere, including the fence around the yard. There were different types of roses in full bloom, holly bushes rushing up the rod iron fence with the "bird of paradise" plants growing freely everywhere.

Christmas Day (December 25, 1997)

Well it's Christmas and all the joy that I hoped for is bursting for a response. We're healthy and happy. I couldn't wait to give Liz the gift I had purposely planned for her and she was quite surprised and grateful. My greatest joy came earlier in the year when I had the desire to do this for her, even though all my plans didn't happen as I had hoped.

When I awakened this morning I remembered the reason for the season, how Jesus came to bring light to a dark world. Just knowing that is enough to rejoice. The weather is so nice with the sun shining with no heavy overcast, birds chirping and I can hear the cars moving at a distance. As I walked out on the patio and sat, I am surrounded by red poinsettias which line the entry way. All the signs of Christmas are present and all I can say is *"God Thank you, for I am so grateful for the giving of your son, Jesus."*

Dad called to wish us a merry Christmas and to see how mom was. After speaking to Mom, Liz and Kendra, he asked to speak to me. In our conversation, he then told me that it was best that mom returned to Omaha with me to live indefinitely. I tried to understand what he was saying, but I did not comprehend. Then he said, if she came back, he would have her put into a home. As those words came through the phone, numbness embraced my body ... my life is about to change again. I don't remember what the conversation was between my sister and I—all I remember was the hurt feeling, being confused, and so many unanswered questions. Not knowing that this was the beginning of a new experience ... a new chapter in my life.

Our return flight was good, just lots of questions that need answers and problems that need solutions. There were decisions to be made regarding Mom's well-being. No one's life changed but mine which was nothing compared to the life of my dear Mother. As I began to ponder things over in my thoughts, I can easily recall all the sacrifices my mother made for me and my children ... how there were times she would just give me a few dollars because she wanted to. All the times she baby sat; all the prayers she prayed for me and my family.

New Year's Eve

New Year's Eve night has always been spent in church for as long as I can remember and tonight is no exception. Mom is here with me, which gives me a sense of joy, knowing that she is here and safe.

From the corner of my eye, I notice how she diligently looks for the scriptures as they are recited and struggles to follow along. I am attentive as she sings, making beautiful music to the Lord and it sounds so good to me. As it gets closer to midnight, I begin to pray, *"Here I am Lord, at the door of 1998 not really knowing, but believing I will cross over into the New Year and answers to my many questions will be revealed."*

3

OUR JOURNEY: WALKING DAILY WITH GOD AND EACH OTHER

o o o o o o o o o o o o o o o o o o o o o o o o o o o o o o o o o o o
"Walk with me Lord, Walk with me; While I am on this tedious journey, I want you Jesus to walk with me."

—*Unknown, old gospel song*

Early morning weekends and late evenings, Mom and I would sit on the front porch to capture the cool breezes during the hot summer months. Mom would spend most days there in the swing, looking at the passing cars and getting up when she'd hear voices of people as they walk by. One of the great things about living in the inner city is the constant noise of people interacting, barking dogs, and the noise. You actually see and hear people and not just see the back of their cars going into the garages as I had experienced living in the suburbs for a number of years.

There would be times Mom would just sit and cry because of the confusion she was experiencing. At times I would sit down and cry with her, for my heart was broken to see her so sad, as the periods of depression continued to escalate. It was a few summers before during one of her visits to Omaha, that she tried to explain what was going on with her, how she wasn't ready to move to Alabama and that it was a mistake. She didn't want to leave her children and grandchildren. She was not happy. In every sense, we were all she had to hold on to. We were very important to her and moving only brought separation and loneliness. Nevertheless she agreed to relocate with the hope of moving to Brewton, Alabama, which was approximately twenty-five miles from where she and Dad had lived and gave birth to us three children. Also it would be near her sister Ruby. They were very close since their families both lived in Omaha prior to moving back to Alabama. Mom was very disappointed in not being able to move to Brewton, but was happy about her new home in Evergreen.

Friends, In the Time of Need

After returning from California, settling in was very difficult the first few months. Since I had to go to work and arrangements had not yet been made with regard to what she would do during the day, I'd take her over to Mother Chaney's or Mother Conway who were dear friends of my mom, both who are older than she. She even spent one day with our Pastor and wife, Elder & Mother Parker, who were very helpful in the transition as were many of our family and friends.

In the beginning I was hesitant to call on all my resources, I guess I really didn't know how people would react, but soon it became necessary. Folk would always say if you need me, just call me. My thoughts and personal experience in the past had been these are only words until they are put into action. Everyone I asked was so receptive and willing to help.

Puzzling Statement (January 14, 1998)

This morning as we were eating grapefruit for breakfast, mom said "I remember when I didn't like grapefruit, and then I started eating them." I don't know where this statement came from, since I have always known her to eat grapefruit. There were many statements made of this kind, it was like she was trying to enlighten me about herself. I just wish I had started taking more notes of her conversations than her actions; I would have learned more about her, her likes and dislikes.

When You don't know what to do, pray (January 25, 1998)

Today was a strange day … so many things had transpired, but it ended with me going into Mom's room and telling her to cry out to God. As she began to pray in Jesus name, I joined in with her for I am looking for a miracle where God restores her memory and relieve her of all this depression and sadness. I believe that she is God's child. Although we prayed until we thought God heard us, I now realize that all we pray for is not in God's perfect plan.

The Friendship Program

It was through the Alzheimer's Association that I obtained most of my information about this facility which was a blessing. Mom's daily attendance here allowed her to keep a sense of freedom and self-worth. She maintained her social skills—they had crafts, music, dance, games, and little outings. When it was ceramic day, they made sure she helped in the set up or at meal time allow her to assist in table setting and food preparation.

I didn't know it then but transportation was going to be our biggest hurdle. We had tried Shared Mobility which was a paid transportation company for individuals who needed special assistance. Other options were sought due to the morning start time at the center and also, there was always a different driver which cased a problem for mom. As friendly as she was, she was not getting in a van with any strangers. Later arrangements were made for the Friendship van to pick her up. Again there was a timing issue. The van started dropping her off at our house; she would unlock the door and go right in. I would be almost right behind her, never leaving her alone more than 10–15 minutes. Then the challenge came when the only solution was to drop her off at the center and pick her up in the evenings.

March 8, 1998

It's amazing how mom can sit for an hour looking at the same papers, over and over. Is she reading and trying to comprehend? What are her thoughts and feelings right now? We had notice a few years prior how she would circle or underline words and/or sentences. Was she rehearsing what she read, or noting important items to remember?

March 16, 1998

Today I noticed that even though Mom is aware of when she does something wrong, she gets loud and defensive; displays anger at her own actions. It hurts her when she can't do the right thing.

Good Friday (April 10, 1998)

This was a holiday for me and it was a wonderful day to be off work. The weather could not have been more perfect. I was going to take advantage of the day by completing some of the tasks previously started and had no time to finish. I dropped Mom off at the Friendship Program, a daycare for seniors. She had been going there on a daily basis for about two months. I was to pick her up after lunch and maybe go shopping.

Just before leaving to pick her up, I received a call from the Friendship Program asking if I or someone else had picked mom up. Usually, if one of my children or my brother was to pick her up, I would let them know in advance. Also, when I picked her up I made sure we exit the front entrance door so that people in the front office would know I was taking her.

My response to the caller was that no one had picked her up. They indicated that they had things under control … I was already on my way. When I arrived, everyone was looking for her, going up and down the surrounding neighborhoods hoping to maybe get a glance of her in the distance. The center had no communication with the van drivers; therefore, they were also waiting for return of the afternoon vans thinking perhaps she had gotten on one of them without the driver's knowledge. If an individual got on the van by mistake, they were brought back to the facility—Mom had unsuccessfully tried this on several occasions. With the return of each van, there was no mom but still hope until the last one came in. The authorities were called and I then called my brother and eldest son. When my son arrived, most of the searchers had returned and the police had put out an alert. He then asked if we had searched east of the facility. The response was no because we didn't believe she would have crossed any of the busy and dangerous streets. One of the searchers came back and indicated a neighbor lady said she had seen a lady fitting mom's description saying "she was walking fast as a woman on a mission." My son couldn't just sit around so he set out on his own search mission. He searched areas to the east then proceeded south. He went into the Baker's Grocery store about a mile away and across 72nd Street, one of the busiest streets in Omaha. After giving the manager a description of mom, he turned to call back to the center to find out if she had been found. At that time, a clerk came up to report to the manager about a lady in the check out line with a basket of food and with no money. Now you have to remember she loved to go grocery shopping and Baker's Grocery was very familiar to her.

This was an experience no one should have to go through, but the chances are each Alzheimer patient will experience some level of wandering. While I was out searching, knocking on doors and talking to strangers on the street, all kinds of those thoughts began to flood my mind. Was she okay, had she fallen and injured herself, and God forbid anyone had picked her up for harm. My only consolation was that this same God whom she prayed to when we were growing up—the one who spared her life in a fatal car accident some years ago, is the same God is watching over her right now. I finally decided to go back to the adult care center when I was told of my son's discovery.

May 4, 1998

Life continues, thanks to the Lord as I try to keep a regular schedule for mom and keeping her busy doing little things around the house. It gives her pleasure in helping. Mom saw a new doctor on Tuesday, Dr. Tim Malloy at the University Medical Center. He told me that I needed to learn all I can about the disease, apply for Medicaid, request her medical records from Dr. Barnes in Alabama and get legal guardianship or power of attorney. The information he was giving left me with feelings of fear and caused me to really consider the issues at hand. He also changed her medications by discontinuing the use of Cognex and ibuprofen; then he prescribed Aricept (10mg) and increased her dosage of Procardia.

Later that evening, we were both very tired after returning from the graduation ceremony of my god-daughter ... I tried to help mom to get ready for bed. This was the first time in all my life that I can remember seeing her hostile. It hurt me so bad, my stomach got into knots, and the feeling was the same as those last days living with my ex-husband. It scared me and left me depressed to the point I wanted to retreat into my shell and hide but I prayed instead.

The next morning Mom knew that she had hurt my feelings as it showed in her actions. I have to constantly remind myself that I should not take it personally. All during the day, with every thought of last night, tears filled my eyes, like I was about to burst; my feet were so heavy and I felt so all alone. Even my children don't understand—Oh well! I don't even understand myself. I still believe with all my heart that God can heal this illness that is overtaking my mom.

May 18, 1998

This was a good day for Mom; she kept saying how she enjoyed the people, referring to the Friendship Program. She even told me they had chicken for lunch and had played ball that afternoon. Once again she is communicating with me.

Annual Women's Conference (May 24, 1998)

I annually attend a religious women's conference during the last week in May. This year it is being held in Kansas City, Missouri. Mom had never been so this would be an opportunity for her to experience the coming together of women from all over the world. We stayed in the hotel and visited family members that Sunday. After attending the services on Monday night, it was a little much for mother. Being in such close quarters at the hotel, she began to get frustrated, walking into the wall mirror, thinking she was going outside. She was constantly going to the door trying to get out. Before going to bed, we walked up and down the halls until I felt she was tired. After the walk, she did have a restful sleep. But considering everything, the large crowds and being out of her comfort zone, we returned to Omaha the next day.

Unexpected Visitor (July 7, 1998)

My Dad came to visit unexpectedly and I was glad he came. It made mom so happy and he was happy to. I spend lots of my time trying to make others happy. Now I know I got my affection from my mom. She stayed in his presence and he had all her attention. It was a lot of pressure for her, adjusting to having him around after being away from him for more than seven months.

Even though the visit threw her off track it was worth just seeing her happy, smiling, and even laughing. My mom loves her husband but she doesn't like how he makes her feel. One thing Dad said, which is true, was that instead of him and mom growing closer they drifted further apart.

As I observe her around him, I see her trying so hard to be herself; trying to stay focused and respond correctly to his questions. She was well aware that she wasn't well. I look at her and feel so sad for her. She deserves so much more; the sadness on her countenance is sometimes overwhelming. No matter what you say or do the sad expressions and depressed feelings come and go. There are times I want to just take and shake her, try to awaken her from this dream; tell her God is with her. I've never known my mother to yell or loose her temper but there was a first, within the last two months and I am almost 49 years old.

August 9, 1998

It has been three weeks today since my brother brought her home after her last weekend visit with him and his wife. He has not even called to see how she is doing. We have seen him twice at other people's home. ***"Lord, help me to not hold a grudge against him, for something I have no control."*** I know that I am only accountable for my own actions in how I treat her and others, but it bothers me. I now understand the pressure Dad was under going through those changes alone. I am however thankful for today … my mother is physically healthy, still functioning, dressing herself, feeding herself and moving about. She continues to give her testimony and sing songs of Zion at church.

Here I am 10:15 AM sitting in the church parking lot, taking a few moments to relax and meditate. I sent mom in for Sunday school so that I could just take time to regroup and have a little personal time. *"Lord thank you, and what ever is coming my way, you are in control, as you are the source of my strength and I know you will carry me through."*

Class Reunion (August 13, 1998)

My sister, Liz arrived today from Los Angeles. Mom and I both were glad to see her and as always, she was her beautiful self. I look so forward to her visits because each time I learn more about her as an adult. This was our Class reunion weekend, so we came home from the airport and tried to relax. The plan was Mom would stay with Kendra while Liz and I went to the class reunion reception. Well, Kendra was late so we decided to go ahead and take mom with us, which was a mistake. As we walked around and mingled with others, we saw the changes in her mood so we sat down with her, trying to include her in our celebration, introducing her to our friends. But the more we catered to her the more uncomfortable she became. She began to cry tears, expressing her desire to go home. We left early enough to get back to the house before it became very difficult.

August 14, 1998

We got up early this morning readying ourselves to go to breakfast. Joe came by and went also which made Liz happy. Whenever we all can get together, we tried to make the best of it. There was not a lot of moving around during the day because of our evening plans. That evening mom was to stay with Valerie while we attended the rest of the reunion festivities. This was not sitting well with mom; we had to leave her with Kendra until Val picked her up. So off we went to Mahoney State Park for the dinner. Also, several of us ladies were staying over night at the cabin. Hind site is always better than foresight—Alzheimer's disease already leaves the individual with memory loss and insecurity, so when they have safe places or familiar persons, they hold on.

With all the rush I forgot the cake for the picnic and it was too late to return to get it. Liz and I returned the next morning to Omaha to get the cake. When I walked into the house everything seemed okay but I noticed a note on the coffee table. It said that our mom was found by the police wandering in a field near 60th & Hartman around 3:30 AM. She was able to tell them her name and address. However, no one was at home. The officers entered into the house but didn't want to leave her alone. They searched through my personal phone book near the phone and ended up calling Dorothy Williams down the street and took her there. God proved himself again that he cares for his children. When questioned later, Mom says she didn't remember anything accept going to Dorothy's house. She didn't understand why all the commotion.

I didn't even call my brother until after the incident was over. I sometime have the feeling that mom's not really important to him and it may be a man thing, but isn't Love the same no matter what gender? I am reminded of a quote I heard which really made sense, *"a son is a son until he takes a wife, a daughter is a daughter for life."*

Moving Again (September, 1998)

Moving involves loss of an important asset, the familiar environment which has been the setting for many of the patient's stored memories of day to day life. Many AD individuals, especially in the early stages, have remarkably good recall of details such as the floor plan of a house and the arrangement of furniture. Unfortunately, most patients find it difficult if not impossible to learn new information.

Prior to mom coming to live with me on a permanent basis, I had purchased a second home back in December 1997 as an investment. I had hopes of fixing it up and renting it out. After I got off work, mom and I would go over to the house and put in 2–3 hours. Mom would do her thing in the kitchen where she felt most comfortable, sweeping and cleaning. The dust would be flying everywhere, then that was the end of that day since I can't work in dust. Mom was with me most of the time and it was getting hard to work over here. After about fifteen minutes she was ready to go home … I did not leave her home alone much … so I ended up moving. This was in deed hard for her, to again move to a strange place all within a year. I tried to make it as comfortable as possible by completing her room first. When we would be returning home from wherever, I had to constantly tell her we no longer live down the street.

First Trip Back to Alabama (September 19, 1998)

Well here we are airborne, flying to Montgomery, Alabama where I rented a car to drive approximately 75 miles south to Evergreen. Wow, it took awhile to prepare for this trip but here we are. Mom seems okay so far—I can see some excitement about her. She wasn't a problem this morning since there was nothing to pack. While she was sleeping I did it all, along with some housework. In the past if I mentioned going out of town, I'd turn around and she was in her room packing. She would have her suitcase on the bed, taking all the clothes down off the hangers, trying to pack.

When we arrived in Evergreen, Dad was very glad to see us. Mom was somewhat confused, but it didn't take her long to get back into the routine. I wish there was some other way, somehow she could stay here. Even though they have only lived here six years, this is home for her, all her stuff is here, her family. I believe she is the happiest here in Evergreen … I've not seen her shed a tear or seem depressed. She stays in the presence of Dad. I don't know how it is going to be when its time to go and what her reactions will be.

As long as she is catered to, she's not irritated. She knows this is her house. In fact, as I was cleaning the kitchen she told me she could clean her own house and she has been sweeping and sweeping ever since, keeping busy trying to stay focused. She still does not like to be corrected even when she knows she is wrong. She moves freely around the house, even outside as I watch her prunes the flowers, sweep the patio, all the normal things she is use to doing.

Prior to coming to Omaha, the guestroom was possibly the room she retreated to when she wanted to be alone. I think she has a problem with me having my things here. If I am in there and she comes in, she quickly does an about face and seems a little frustrated. So I sort of kept my things in the suitcase over in the corner so as to not give her the impression I'm taking over. Once she was about to rush out and I ask her to come in and sit on the bed; we just talked. I asked her about the little "whatnots" on the wall and how the cool breezes come in this room. It would relax her and she'd say something like, "well dear, guest I need to get up and get busy."

Every morning Dad gets up and goes for a walk, returns and prepares breakfast … cleans the kitchen, sit and watch television. He is pretty much set in his ways and has his set routines. I wonder, did he ever take mom along for the company? Change is often hard when one does not want to deal with the issues at hand. For the most part, he is a loner and mom is a people person but content just being with him. At this age she still wants his attention and approval and there is nothing wrong with that.

The "I Love You" Words

Friday morning mom was a bear—she had been up and down all night, with hardly any sleep and early this morning she was getting up with Dad. She wants so much to please him. She got up and began getting dressed; putting on the same clothes she had on the day before. As I attempted to help her, she became very hostile towards me not wanting my help. I once again explained to her that I was only trying to help her. It is hard for Alzheimer's disease patients to accept the fact that one is trying to help, she even told me "you are not my daughter" which I thought was very cruel of her to say. To be honest, it hurt my feelings and it should not have. She dashed out of the bathroom and went to the breakfast table without her partial in her mouth. She tried to go to the table but just walked around in circles. Sometimes, you have to step back and just wait.

Again, trying to be creative in my actions I was able to get her dressed. Dad told her how good she looked and for the first time I can remember, I heard my Dad tell my mom "I Love You." In my family, this phrase is not taken lightly. When we heard it, we knew it was for real.

After breakfast she was wore out and fell asleep on the couch. I went into the back room to rest and relax. It is times like this that I must find a quiet place to praise and worship God through prayer. My prayer started, ***"Lord, thank you for this time. I realize that things were moving too fast and I am not where I should be, help me to decrease so that you may increase. I can't do this alone. I need your help, lead me in the path I should go. You are my strength and my strong tower."***

September 27, 1998

Here we are again at the airport waiting on our return flight to Omaha. Mom is somewhat confused as usual these days; she thinks that she will return home with Uncle William and Annie. They came along with us to the airport so that Dad would not have to ride back alone. After getting settled in at the airport, they had overbooked the flight and were asking for volunteers to give up their seat and take the evening flight to Atlanta … I always see this as an opportunity but not this trip.

We arrived in Atlanta to find out that our flight was cancelled for whatever reason. The airline put us up in a hotel with no luggage but we managed. Although we had separate beds, we slept together in the same bed. This gave her comfort in knowing that I was right there and also I would hear if she got up out of the bed. I have learned that individuals with AD like to move around at night, both quietly and quickly. I had to be real creative since neither of us had our luggage, just an overnight bag which included her medication and a change of underwear if she had an accident. I guess she is getting accustom to being around me because she was not distraught or scared. Besides her questions, all went well. We flew out the first thing the next morning, first class. We felt special as we looked at each other and began to laugh.

November, 1998

I went to Memphis leaving Mom with my brother and his wife. This was a special trip for me in two ways; my pastor's wife was being installed as the Supervisor of Women in the State of Nebraska and I would again see this special person I met earlier this summer—He is currently living here.

February 25, 1999

I had major surgery and was off work for a few months. The first week of recovery I stayed with my daughter and her family while mom stayed with my brother. During this time, I call the "silent weeks" because I didn't write much, just read a lot.

Los Angeles Trip (April 16, 1999)

Mother and I flew to Los Angeles for my cousin Miesha's wedding. She enjoyed seeing her sister-in-law and other family members. It was not as difficult as I thought it would be, perhaps because Mom has become accustomed to having me around. She didn't let me get too far out of her site.

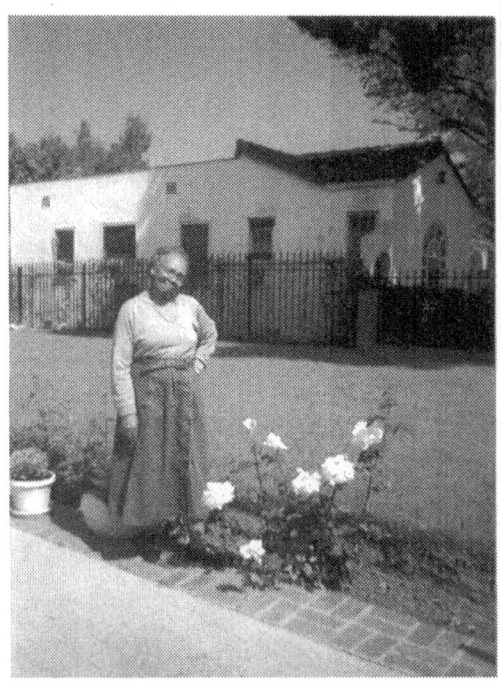

A Rose posing with California roses.

May 14, 1999

My friend from Detroit came to visit for a few days. Mom was very pleasant to my guest but tried to avoid being in the same room with him; she didn't talk much just listened and smiled. Wherever we went, I took mom along with us; I really wanted him to know of my commitment to her. If I had approached that relationship differently, I probably would be happily married today, then maybe not.

May 27, 1999

Today Mom displayed such anger … it was as if she had no space to move or anything to do. She kept saying quietly to herself that I was always telling her what to do and that she was not a child. I am still trying to figure out what is going on.

June 6, 1999

This morning, I came to grips with the question asked often, why me. There is no more why or how come. My mom is how God wants her to be right now. Nothing or no one else can remove her from this point, except God. I pray that if her condition is what is planned for me, let me die before then. I never want to be in this state or want my children to have to endure this hardship. ***"OH GOD, she is so unhappy, angry and unsettled, its beginning to be more frequent now, I don't know if its dad or not. But Lord, in this you are in control. If there is any glory in her condition, so be it. I can only thank you for the times Mom and I shared in earlier years."***

Family Reunion—Omaha, Nebraska (July 4, 1999)

We had family coming from all over the USA. Mom was glad to see everyone and everyone was glad to see her. With all of the activities she remained calm. Her sisters, Mary, Roberta and Ruby helped manage things so she wouldn't be too overwhelmed.

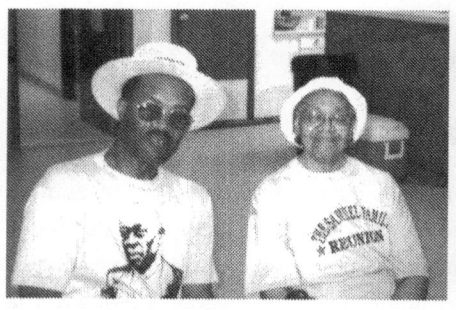
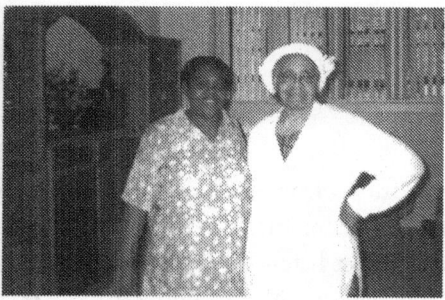

Arnold & Eula at the Samuel Reunion   Eula and her youngest sister, Mary

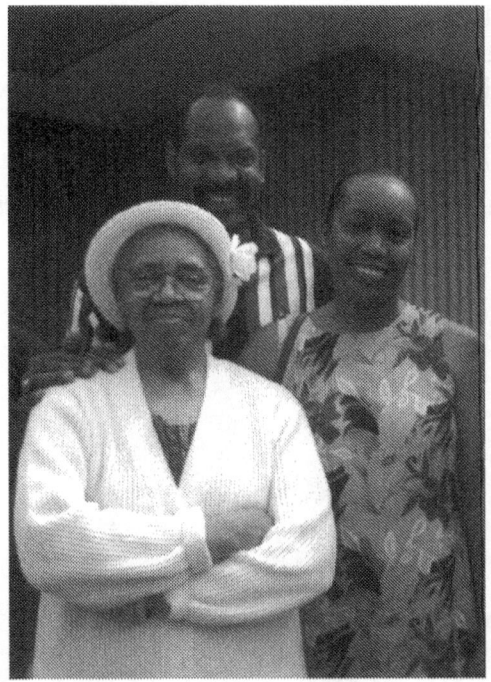

Mom, Joe and Liz

Birthday Celebration

This was a great year for me, I celebrated my 50th birthday. I have always enjoyed making plans for my birthday because I feel each year is a milestone and a time of celebration. I am so blessed to have lived to get to this age.

As a child I suffered with asthma and there were many times I thought I was taking my last breath. I was about the age of 13 when God miraculously healed me of this sickness. I no longer suffer with asthma. I was attending the local business college, where I met an older gentleman in whom I had great compassion. He had such a hard time with asthma; he died of an asthma attack a year after we met—So I celebrate each year.

My friend Joe came from Detroit to help celebrate this special day with me. Even though he had been here before and had met Mom, it was difficult for her having some stranger in the house. She was nice to him, but I could tell she was uncomfortable. It was difficult, but he tried to take my mind off of her condition and the amount of stress I was under.

On Friday we all got dressed for this very special occasion. Mom was so beautiful in her black sequence two-piece attire and she was very attentive to me and my guest. My brother Joe came and picked her up which allowed me time to get dress and pamper myself before I make my grand entrance. It was a great celebration at the downtown Omaha Press Club where more than seventy-five invited guest attended. Also, it was when I officially introduced my special friend to the family.

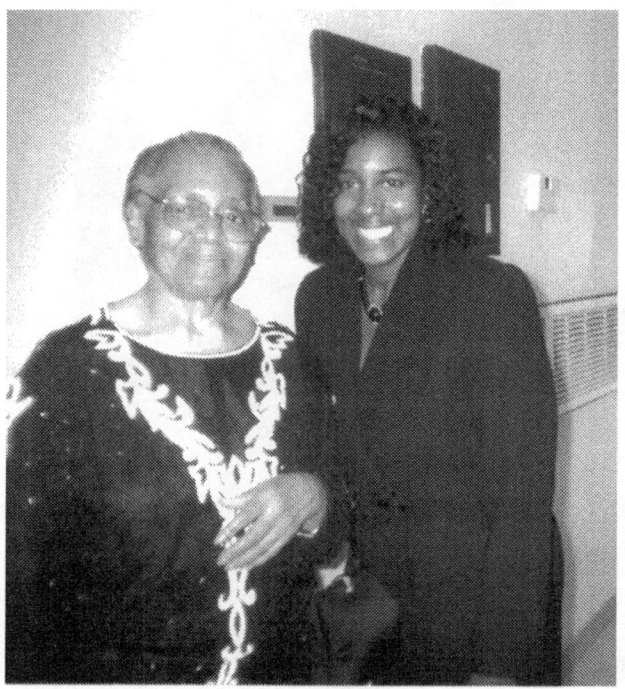

Valarie and Mom at my birthday celebration

It was during this weekend, that I realized I could not share this burden with anyone else. I tried to keep a distant relationship going, but it didn't last as my commitment is here, caring for Mom.

November 19, 1999

"Thank you God, for another day." I've been under the weather the past few days and I realize how difficult it is to care for Mom when I am not feeling well. I remember having similar feelings years ago when I was going through a difficult

marriage and various issues with my youngest son. I am supposed to leave in a few days to spend Thanksgiving in Detroit, but it doesn't look too good; but I desperately need the break.

November 24, 1999

I left for Detroit hoping to have a wonderful time, which I did but bitter sweet memories is all I brought back with me. I have always known that when Christ is not the center of your plans, broken dreams is all that can be. My thoughts were of mom, who stayed with my brother and his wife. Leaving her wasn't getting any easier, but I was learning to let him help more with her care.

Christmas and the Turn of the Century

Mom and I were flying off again to Alabama. After renting a car in Montgomery, Mom and I arrived in Evergreen about 1:00 PM. Dad as always, was glad to see us. He had decorated the outside of the house with all the beautiful lights around the edge of the roof and the trees nearest the house. He had gone into the woods and cut down this great evergreen tree and put out the Christmas decorations for me and mom to decorate inside.

He still has the same routine every morning; he goes for a walk and returns, prepares breakfast, clean the kitchen and that's it. He watches television and on occasion he'd go visit the sick or some of his sisters or brothers near by. A lot of it has to do with his physical health. Dad had worked hard all those many years, providing for his family and now has problems with his back and with his heart. When there is company, he enjoys laughing and talking about sports and can talk about politics until the subject is changed.

Our stay was only a few days, which is shorter than usual. We had heard so much about the turn of the century and with all of the uncertainty, so our plan was to return to Omaha before the turn of the century. Of all the times we had come to visit, this was one of most difficult, mom really didn't want to leave dad. In later conversations with Dad, he said she had pleaded with him to let her stay, telling him she would be okay.

Happy New Year (January 2, 2000)

This morning, mom wouldn't eat breakfast so I fed her; its funny how she holds her mouth open like a little kid. She really didn't eat much dinner either, just cornbread and veggies. I think she may have been missing home and wondering where Hick was.

January 3, 2000

Some mornings were better than others. Today began on a happy note as she allowed me to photo her before breakfast. I thought she look cute with her new short hair style.

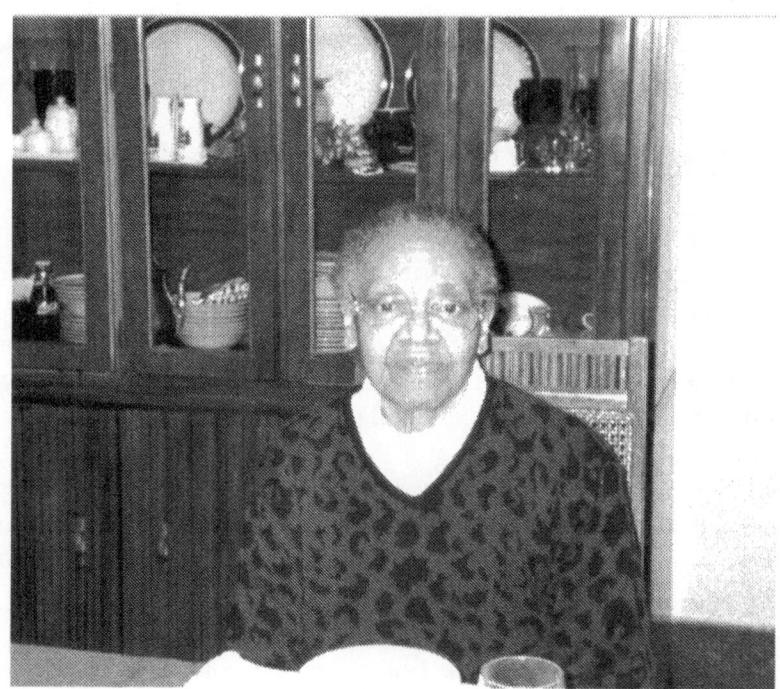

"Quiet Morning"

It was a good day. I picked Mom up after work and we took a little detour home. We pulled up outside Viola's house, one of Mom's first cousins. She was outside and immediately mom said "that's Mutt." I asked her to verify and she said "Mutt, Viola" as if to refresh my memory or to let me know she knew who she was. They were glad to see each other. And I was happy that she recognized her. We visited with her for awhile, not getting out of the car, and then we left assuring Viola that we would do this more often. There were a couple of days that the Friendship program was closed–Mom would spend the day with her talking, laughing and reminiscing. They grew up together being two brother's children. That meant so much, to know that family was available in time of need. I wanted to make sure that I was not taking those family ties for granted.

Visit With Mom's Caseworker (January 4, 2000)

This morning I met with mom's Medicare caseworker, Joanne Whitcre. She spoke of her mom who also has Alzheimer's and is in a nursing home. Her Dad was the caregiver and it got to be too much for him and became too stressful for him. There were some encouraging words given as she stressed that I should not feel guilty about seeking out future plans for Mom. I needed to check with nursing homes that would allow for temporary adult care or respite for a smoother transition. I indicated to her that at this point, I don't know how I would feel having someone come into the home. Although it would be better for me, then I could then care for her in the evenings.

Great Routines Equal Great Results

Each morning, I go into her room saying good morning … asking how she is doing. Over and over here reply would be "pretty good" and I would respond "pretty good is hard to beat sometime" and a big smile would come upon her face. Now it is hard for her to form those two simple words … there are times she really tries to talk and the words are not there, but I can make out her phrases. I just agree or say "for real" then she will continue, using hand motions, etc. If I didn't get her up, she would probably stay in bed. Anyway, I get her to set up and rub her back and shoulders. I massage her as if someone was massaging me. When I ask if it feels good, she will respond "yes." The mind works harder to respond with an answer so it is best to keep it simple. Other times she tunes me out as the old folks say, get a deaf ear.

May 8, 2000

Here it is a year later; life's surroundings are continuously changing. Mom is steady loosing weight. Is it her mind that won't tell her to eat? I fed her again on yesterday. She is misplacing her eye glasses more frequently and the night before she had taken out her upper partial and put it under her pillow.

She has been experiencing difficulty in making it to the bathroom at night. When she awaken in the mornings she is drenched, bed and all. I purchased her a porta-pot for her room, thinking that if she saw it she'd use it. It worked for awhile, and then she started using the floor in the closet. I began to schedule getting her up during the night, with one eye open and one closed. There were times it was convenient and times when she wouldn't do a thing.

June 24, 2000

Sitting here at the Life Care Center, I am waiting for an interview about the possibility of respite and/or long term care here. I began to observe people coming and going. After seeing all of these elderly people, I wonder what is the average age, what part of the country are they from and where are their children if any. I over heard one man saying to another, "Is that woman a loose again," then I observed the expressions of one lady's son and daughter who were saying good bye.

July 21, 2000

Well it's been almost a week since Dad returned to Alabama. Harvey my eldest son drove him home and should be coming back this evening. Mom has been having a hard time adjusting to him being gone. At first; she would be looking for Dad when we came in from the Friendship Program, looking behind me and around corners. Several times she'd get up and go into the kitchen or to the porch, never asking where he was, just looking.

Although she is having some good days, I believe that something is wrong with her bladder. She is always drenched in the morning. Since she has begun wearing Depends, I make sure that I always carried extras in the car. She likes carrying a purse or something in her hand, so I purposely put a Depend, paper/pencil and peppermint candy in a bag for her to carry.

August 20, 2000

We had gone over to the rental house to drop off some items. As we were standing near the car talking to the neighbor, Mr. and Mrs. Morgan, mom just collapsed. I was able to catch her before her head could hit the ground. We just had her lay there until the rescue squad came. When they arrived, she had regained consciousness. The medics kept asking her questions and I kept saying she doesn't understand. After getting their attention, I told them of her condition so that they would understand some of her actions. Mom was not about to be restrained so she put up a good fight. They were able to restrain her and took her to emergency as I followed in my car. They kept her over night for observation and some test which resulted in her having symptoms of a mini stroke. AD patients have a history of these kinds of episodes and the doctor says there will be more. She was released and we came home.

September 9, 2000

This was going to be a busy day so I got up exceptionally early, took my bath and just pampered myself. Since Mom had to run with me all day, I let her sleep until she was ready to awake. Our last stop for the day was the beauty shop. There were times we would be getting our hair done at the same time, but now she has a problem with other folks doing her hair.

Before getting started, I asked if she had to use the restroom, she says no. But past experience lets me know that she should be ready to go and she is looking wet. We go into the restroom, get cleaned up and dispose of her undergarment. I had no change for her and figured she wouldn't have to go again before we got home. Then less than 15 minutes when she got up, she was soaking wet, there was a sense of embarrassment for me. Those that were in beauty shop were very attentive and concern.

We got home and it was like retaliation towards a child for acting up—I was upset with her, and it didn't set with her either. While trying to get her situated in the bathroom, she went through her ritual "get your tail out of here, I'm going to kill you, on and on. She tried to hit me but I grabbed both her hands and held her. I was all too conscious of the moment ... I just looked at her not saying a word, and after getting her attention, she calms down. This morning I had already prayed and bound the devil, then to have the day to end like this ... no way Hosea.

November 30, 2000

On a work related road trip to northern California, I was sitting in the café surrounded by old retired males, talking about today's news, stock, the fact that we have no president, credit cards, computers ... what they didn't talk about. These are times when I think of how my mom was *robbed of the rest of her life*, the enjoyment of growing old gracefully, sitting back and talking about the day. I believe that if her situation was different, she would be sitting with her friends talking about the same subjects over a cup of coffee. She had always kept up with the local and national news. She would have been one of those seniors going back to school to learn the computers to enhance her great secretarial skills.

December 7, 2000

Today, I have been feeling strange, physically feel bad. My brother came over to visit and as always, I love to see him and to know how he is doing. I only have one brother and I want to see him happy. I know that we all have our own issues, but I just wish he would insist on helping more.

Mom is sleeping longer and it's getting hard at times to get her up in the mornings. Lord I wish I could sleep like that, but I just have too much to do. When I do lie down, I can think of 150 things that need to be done, so I toss and turn all night.

December 31, 2000

I am discussed and don't want to fight with mother's spirit today. I want to walk out and leave her, but I remember the commitment I made to her. I continue to tell myself this is how God wants it to be!

Appointment with the Caseworker (January 4, 2001)

Another year has past, with my mornings getting a little more complicated. At first, Mom didn't want to get up and she didn't want to eat so I had to feed her breakfast. Another rush morning—I was scheduled to meet her caseworker at 8:30 AM, and my doctor's appointment was at 10:30 AM.

I met with mom's caseworker Joanne Whitaker, who is very nice and seem very understanding. I really wanted to talk about what other alternatives I have regarding the care of mom. Joanne was eager to hear how things were going since our last visit a year ago. I shared with her some of the ordeals or should I say the good times and the bad. Top of my list was how it is getting hard for me to get her up in the mornings, she wants to sleep, and I want and need to go to work. Nothing concrete was decided but she again gave me some ideas and encouraged me to take care of myself. I have heard this over and over and I try to … I have no personal life so nothing is lacking there. I oft times sit and think about what I would be doing if I was not caring for mom. Most time, nothing comes to mind that is more important than her care.

We did decide that I would check into various nursing facilities that have an adult day care where Mom could attend occasionally and gradually become a resident. It is inevitable that the time for institutionalization is approaching. Last summer I did not think that she would be with me this long; in fact I was telling my daughter that I was keeping her until the 1ˢᵗ of the year … which is now.

Mom was giving me such a hard time; it's like she knew it and wasn't giving me any slack after my vacation back in October to Jamaica where I did get a lot of rest and relaxation, a new boost. My sister came from California to stay with mom while I was gone. This was good for her too. That week, I believe she learned a lot about mom and the care she requires. Do we ever really know a situation until we experience it; life is the best teacher. I have always learned something from my sister when I am in her presence. I love visiting her in California, because of what I would learn or experience, something new I could take back home to use, put into action, say, or wear. Her singleness was exciting to me, being an old married lady back then. Now I know single life is like married life, it is what you make of it.

Another Year has Past (January 12, 2001)

As I set across from mom, she seemingly not caring about anything, plays with her hands, looking at the wall trying not to look at me by avoiding eye contact. I wonder how long this will go on.

January 15, 2001

Sunday was a good day. Mom really participated in the service, clapping her hands, singing and listening to the preacher, as if she understood what was being said. Later that evening, Joe and his wife, Loraine came over to visit.

January 19, 2001

It is amazing how she can stand for an hour in the same spot, so long as her hands are moving. I can ask her to sit and she will, as if she is waiting for instructions on what to do. I notice that when she has to go to the bathroom, she starts pacing, possibly trying to locate the restroom.

Her physical make up is changing so, a lot of her muscle fat is leaving, her arms and legs are so small, it is as if she is shrinking, can that be. I never knew she was so short. I do remember her always wearing high heals and hats that probably added height. She had always been a healthy lady averaging 175–200 pounds. Now she weighs less than 135 lbs. Sitting looking into her face, all the pain that I see and then she can crack a smile that removes all the strain. She holds her head down a lot and won't look me in the eye. Sometimes when she is agitated, I put my hands on her chin to get her to look at me and I talk to her, slowing her down, and then she calms down.

Battles No One Can Win

Mom was very regular and we never had problems until now. After we arrived home, she would go directly to the bathroom on the first floor or even go upstairs. As time progressed, I had to direct her to the bathroom and she would handle herself well. Then she began getting off schedule and had an accident, which was the beginning of many. When this happened, we went up stairs to get cleaned up because the bathroom on the first floor was not large enough for the both of us. As time passed, it began to get pretty bad as her angry outburst escalated. There have been times when it was all out holy war. She would fight like a wild person, which was funny at times because she did not know how to fight. It was not at me that she was angry, but at what was happening to her.

In a quest to find out how far she would go, there was one occasion that I did let her strike me, I mean she tried to punched me out, scratched at me, and even bit me. I made sure that I guarded my face and that any large objects were out of sight. I was quite in control as I told her to get all the anger out. My thinking was that if she rid this anger, there would be peace. But I really knew this was the beginning of many battles to come and I stay strong for both our sakes. After she was wore out, she returned to her room and closed the door. If I was tired then, what state am I in now?

There were many days after that I didn't know what to do. I was constantly on my knees asking God for direction. In one sitting as I was mediating, I believe it was the spirit of God that said *"You have to care for her, like you enjoy it, not as a task or heavy burden; but as it is a blessing."* The situation didn't get better, but I began to handle situations differently. From this, I have learned about myself, about my mother, about my family and extended family and about a disease no one ever talked about in depth. I remember old folks saying phrases like *"so and so done went crazy,"* which was not the case, they had a disease no one could explain.

Church Services

She has such joy in attending church as in the past. This is where she felt most comfortable as the months passed. There would be times I would want to leave early and she would not budge. She'd get her shout on and you knew what song she was going to sing, "Have you tried Jesus." As the disease progressed, she'd sing the same song every service. Sometimes she would forget the words and look over at me to help her out, and of course I would. Then, it got to the point where she'd ask me what song to sing, if she was called upon the sing a solo. Pastor was good at keeping her involved by doing just that. I remember the last time she sang a solo at a Friday night service. She got up and could not think of a song to sing so I went up and made a suggestion and sang with her.

February 5, 2001

On the way home I didn't feel like cooking dinner and didn't feel like stopping to pick up anything, I just came on home and forced myself to cook. Mom is in somewhat of a good mood. She was dry and willingly used the bathroom. Usually when she comes in, if she is wet it causes her to be very irritable and quiet. Joe called indicating that he was coming over. He brought a beautiful picture of him and Lorraine. In our conversation, he asked if we had plans for Sunday and I told him that I would be out of town. He didn't ask about where mom would be and I didn't say. I wasn't ready to tell him about the nursing home and my decision, but I did. I don't know how he felt, but right then it was not my concern. I'm not giving up but it's like no relief, I have not learned to use the various services available to me and there are many. My sister, Liz must have sensed something because right after Joe left, she called. I ended up telling her that the date would be around Mother's day; that I had not totally decided. I could tell in her voice the sadness but she reassured me that, I had done all I could.

February 25, 2001

As I observe Mom; she is weaker these days, but she still keeps going. This strong soldier, during these cold days of winter, still gets up, only a little slower and needs more coaxing. I feel guilty and don't like getting her up, but I need to go to work. But we'd get dressed, bundled up and out the door we went.

February 26, 2001

Her love for music is alive and well … Her little fingers get to bouncing, patting her feet as she begins to hum. She hums more and is still able to harmonize, but sings very little. When you're talking on the phone, she is responding, is it that we talk to her differently?

March 2, 2001

The Friendship Program reported that Mom was very tired today. When we arrived home I prepared dinner and she ate very well. Two of my grandsons, DJ and Myles were over for a visit. When it was bedtime, we all went into Mom's room and had prayer (DJ recited the Lord's Prayer). The boys seem to get joy out of helping put Granny to bed; pulling the cover up over her, rubbing her head, kissing her and saying "good night Granny."

Time of Forgiveness (March 14, 2001)

Harvey Sr. to whom I had been married for twenty three years and now divorced, came over to speak with mom … it was so touching, not him saying what he did but the letter he read to her. Mom had written to him in 1984 at a time when he was going through some rough times, which caused him to hurt a lot of folks who loved him; mom was one of them. Back then if she couldn't say what needed to be said, she put it in writing. In her letter she indicated that God had reveal to her about his ministry and what he needed to do. That he was the wall between God and the church growing, he needed to get home straight first. All of which was true and I guess now he needed to bring closure to the animosity he held towards her for a number of years. I never knew about the letter until now. She listened attentively but I don't know if she understood but at least he felt relieve or forgiven.

March 15, 2001

This was a blessed day also, my son in law Doug, had found some of Hope's things among his and left them out for her to discard. Going through what seen some old items, she discovered a letter from Mom dated back in 1994. I believe it was for her to know who her grandma was and I thank God because she needed to know that her "granny" loves her very much.

Her love for music remains as her little fingers get to bouncing and her feet still pats at the sound of the beat; she hums more, but sings little. When you are talking on the phone, she is all in your conversation, responding as if I am talking to her.

Last Trip Home (March 26–31, 2001)

I took Mom back to Alabama for what I believed to be her last visit. We were accompanied by one of my god-daughters, Tasha and her daughter. I did all the driving and Tasha basically helped with mom keeping her busy and entertained. Everything went well with the weather being great for driving. Mom was for the most part quiet. I tried to make frequent stops so she wouldn't get irritable. We spent the night in Paducah, Kentucky where she slept well and I slept with one eye open. Even though she had not roamed in awhile, it is a habit now to be on the alert. In the morning, I made sure she took a relaxing bath, had a balanced breakfast and took all her pills. We were again on our way.

When she saw her sisters and brothers, her facial expressions indicated that she recognized them, especially Aunt Ruby and her brother Roosevelt. Aunt Mary and my cousin Dorothy were the only ones who really acknowledged the reason for this trip. We had all gathered at Aunt Ruby's house, sitting and enjoying one another's company. As we began to prepare to leave, Aunt Mary hugged me and held me tight, saying "take care of Baby for me and do what you can." We both began to cry for she knew the road I was about to travel. Although she is only a few years older than I, she had been down this road more times than once, caring for my grandmother, grandfather and Aunt Hattie Mae.

We visited my dad's brother, Uncle Lois who was very happy to see her. Mom had cared for his wife for a couple of years before being institutionalized. She had all the symptoms of AD but I don't know if she was ever diagnosed. When we were about to leave, Uncle Lois jumped up and went into the other room and came out with a $100 bill. The expression on his face was a sight to behold as he placed it in her hands with joy. She took it without hesitation saying thank you—she definitely remembered the value of money. I'm sure she remembered all the times in the past when he had put some change in her hand for helping care for Aunt Hattie. Uncle Lois knew where she has been and what lies ahead. It had been a year since Aunt Hattie Mae died after being in the nursing home a few years. Prior to that he cared for her at home, watching and enduring all the changes she was going through—trying to explain to her when she didn't seem to understand. I remember one incident where she had said something offensive and he said "Now Hattie, you know that was not the right thing to say" and I am sure there were times he had to raise his voice, but I never heard it.

It was really rough for me knowing in my heart that it was my last time bringing her home and it had an affect on Dad as well. I tried to imagine her never coming back here to sleep in her own bed, prune her flowers and say this is home, tears began to fill my eyes because it is true. I tried to make her as comfortable as possible; keeping my stress level down and pacing myself so I can help her more. If she wanted to sit, I let her set, if she went outside, I'd watch from the window.

Our return trip to Omaha went well; my dad returned with us. The morning of the second day of our trip, we had stopped to get a quick breakfast at McDonalds. After getting everyone settled, I went across the way to get gas. When I returned, Dad was returning from the restroom and going outside to stretch his legs. As I was waiting for Mom to finish eating, Tasha and her daughter returned to the van. At that point, maybe is where it all started. I can't recall what set it off but Mom wouldn't get up from the table so that we could leave. She wanted to sit and that was okay for awhile. The mistake I made was trying to help her up from the table, she started pulling back. Embarrassment came over me when a gentleman was holding the door open for us while I pulled her out. I held tight to her arm as we walked to the van. As we approached the van, she tried to walk off, so rather than getting in on the driver's side I had to catch her and even physically put her into the van. Dad didn't know what happened, and didn't know how to help. After getting her in, he asked "Eula Mae why you acting like that." She responded with "acting like what." After about an hour she was still upset, which left everyone else on edge but there were no more incidents. The remaining drive was long and quiet.

April 17, 2001

We arose early as usual and got dressed. Mom was not irritable but disoriented; we were unable to get her partial back in after cleaning. Usually I would do hand motions to show her how to take her partial out and put it back in, but that didn't work this time. She had no problem brushing her lower teeth and using mouthwash.

Administering her medication was beginning to be a problem. Where she once would just put them in her mouth and swallow, now she holds them in her mouth. I've noticed that a pill would be on her plate or under the napkin. So now I have to make sure she swallows them before I walked away. It was breakfast and off to the Friendship program, without her partial. Still not able to function well enough to put her partial in her mouth, she had to eat dinner without it.

Putting her to bed was no problem tonight. In fact, I sat in the chair next to her bed and laid on her shoulder, I could see her smile. The maternal instinct is still there ... I rubbed her hair, her ears, her forehead as I began thinking how this phenomenon woman brought such a phenomenon woman into this world. I can see so much of her in me.

A Scary Call (April 23, 2001)

Today I received a call from Immanuel Fontennelle indicating they had an opening for Mom. It caught me off guard and I didn't know what to say. The caller informed me that I need to respond in a week—the feelings are unexplainable right now, sitting at my desk at work, all I could think was *"no, no, no."* I panic and responded to the caller *"I need to but I am not ready."* How dare they call me and tell me "it is time." Why was I so offended? I placed her name on the list, no one forced me. What happens when the others call? After coming to terms with the situation, which seem longer than it was, I asked that she be placed at bottom of list. It was very painful for me the rest of the work day. When I got home I hugged her and thought today is not the day. I had cut back on Depakote; she is more irritable than usual, literally shaking when I put her to bed.

Friends Here Today, Gone Tomorrow (4-29-01)

This was a most devastating day. Cheryl, a co-worker called to tell me about a close friend and co-worker, Nadine McWilliams, had died before day. As I dropped to the floor I began to yell. Dad came into my room and tried to comfort me. All I could say was that we had just had lunch that Friday to plan for my daughter's baby shower. It seems almost impossible, how could this be. Mom was undisturbed by my actions as she was still asleep.

May 7–12, 2001

The first week of this month, I attended the International Women's Convention, held in Birmingham, Alabama. This was a religious retreat for me, full of inspiration and plenty of rest.

Since Dad was here, I had asked him to take care of her while I was gone. I guest he didn't feel comfortable doing so. He was also very uncomfortable with the idea that I had asked Tasha to come and take care of her. If I didn't think she could handle Mom, I would have never asked her. Tasha was a young lady who found herself homeless and pregnant; she had lived with me for two years prior to mom coming to stay. After she gave birth to her daughter and got back on her feet, she moved out. Even after she moved, she would still come and sit with Mom while I ran errands. Long story short, I ended up taking mom to Maple Crest nursing home for respite, which she has been many times before in the Alzheimer unit. She did very well. It was then that I asked the home to schedule her for the third week in June for respite while I was to be working out of town and possibly for long-term stay. When I did that, it was sort of a relief.

Morning Observations

Most mornings, there is a rush to get things done, causing me to be late for work everyday about 10–15 minutes. I could get mom up earlier, but guilt sets in, she has worked all those years, this should be a time to sleep in. But I do believe if it were not for her getting up and out each morning she would be less active that she is now. There were some mornings I would have to assist her in eating, even feed her which makes me late for work.

She can no longer dress herself or even pull up her depends and when I try to put on her socks, she literally holds her feet down. Don't know why, perhaps it's a way of saying "I m still here and having feelings;" she doesn't want to surrender that sense of independence, which she shouldn't have to. There are times that I would let her sit on the toilet for an extended time, giving her time to relax. Today, I took advantage of this time by asking her a few questions that Dr. Malloy would ask during her visits:

What is your name	Eula Mae
How old are you Eula Mae	could not answer
What is your husband's name	no answer
Do you have any children	yes
How many children do you have	four
Where were you born	could not answer

She is still very easily distracted as she pulls her hair on the left side and constantly digs in her nose. She is having less bowl movements which causes me concern and her hips seem to be getting bigger which may be part of her family traits. We call them the "Samuel Hips" because most of my folk on her side of the family have them sooner or later.

It is so hard for me to sit down and evaluate mom, where do I start? Do I ask questions she can't answer verbally—she only mutters, trying to get something out which I can not understand. I've made the decision now it's hard to move forward. It's like every thing is okay now, but its not, I am getting more frustrated and short tempered.

May 25, 2001

We went to the hospital for the birth of baby Nolan, my fifth grandson. Since no prior plan had been made, Mom accompanied me to the hospital. She was very tired but it was hard to keep her down. She stayed alert as long as she could but we eventually had her lay down on the sofa, where she finally went to sleep.

May 31, 2001

Mom returned home from the Friendship Program without her upper partial in her mouth. I had the center look for it but to no avail, so now she has to eat softer foods and learn how to use her gums with some help from her lower front teeth. I guess what made me most angry is the fact that she came in and sat with Dad until I came. He had not noticed it until I said something. When I first walked in and saw her at the table, I notice it. It is possible that I have programmed myself to pay attention to her and her needs.

June 4, 2001

I had an appointment to meet with Carol Braum at Maple Crest today. Although Mom had respite there on many occasions, she wanted to go over the procedures for admission into the nursing facility. There were applications and forms to be complete.

June 14, 2001

Mom still recognizes my dad and her mood still changes when he comes in her presence. Today, she is humming which is a sign of joy. She plays a lot with her fingernails and continues to cross her legs at the ankles. She turns her head as she becomes aware of me staring at her.

June 22, 2001

I took a half day vacation from work to do some shopping and prepare Mom's room at Maple Crest for her arrival on tomorrow. This evening has been exceptionally hard for me. We had cake at the Friendship program as a thank you for the care given to mom and celebrating her last day there. I don't know if she realized what was going with all the attention she was getting. Although she was excited, I did notice some expressions on her face indicating some confusion.

4

ALZHEIMER'S DISEASE: AN UNKNOWN THIEF ROBS AGAIN

o o o o o o o o o o o o o o o o o o o o o o o o o o o o o o o o o o

"I fear I am not in my perfect mind, me thinks I should know you, and know this man, yet I am doubtful; for I am mainly ignorant what place this is; and all the skill I have remembers not these garments; nor I know not where I did lodge last night. Do not laugh at me."

—*Shakespear Play; King Lear, Act IV, Scent 7*

This disease is named after Dr. Alois Alzheimer, a German doctor who in 1906, noticed changes in the brain tissue of a woman who had died of an unusual mental illness. He found abnormal clumps (now called amyloid plaques) and tangled bundles of fibers (now called neurofibrillary tangles). It was his research that brought attention to the changes in brain tissue. Today, these plaques and tangles in the brain are considered signs of Alzheimer's disease (AD). Scientist do not yet fully understand what causes AD and concludes there probably is not one single cause, but several factors that affect each person differently. Age however is the most important known factor.

Alzheimer's is incurable and irreversible. It results in progressive brain damage, slowly destroying memory and thinking skills. It changes the way a person acts, thinks and responds—it seriously affects a person's ability to carry out daily activities. The time span is usually seven years but can last 2–20 years. Although AD is the most common form of dementia, most of us had never heard much about AD until the early 80's. It was in 1983 President Reagan designated

November as Alzheimer's Disease Month. This was before he developed the disorder. It was his hope to raise public awareness about this devastating illness.

According to an 2006 article in the Alzheimer's Association-Midlands Chapter newsletter, Alzheimer's will become a 21st century epidemic as it begins its assault on millions of baby boomers within the next 10 years.

- Medicare spends $91 billion a year on care for people with Alzheimer's disease. That cost will double to approximately $189 billion by 2015.

- Medicaid spends at least $21 billion on Alzheimer's long-term nursing home care, a figure expected to hit $27 billion by 2015.

- Alzheimer's disease costs American businesses $61 billion a year in lost productivity of caregivers in the work force and associated health care expenses.

Symptoms, Diagnosis and Medications

AD begins slowly with symptoms of mild forgetfulness, which can easily be confused with aged-related memory change. Please don't get alarmed if you can identify with this, most people with mild forgetfulness do not have AD. In the early stage of AD, a person may have trouble remembering recent events, activities, or the names of familiar people or things.

Today, the only definite way to diagnose AD is to find out whether there are plaques and tangles in the brain tissue, which is through an autopsy, an examination of the body done after a person dies. Therefore, doctors can only make a diagnosis of "possible" or "probable" AD while the person is alive.

On July 3, 1996, I met with mom's physician Dr. Stanley Barnes there in Evergreen, Alabama. I shared some of her symptoms and my concerns. He then ordered several test for her after which she was diagnosed as possible Alzheimer's disease.

AD is not curable but its symptoms are treatable. The Federal Drug Administration (FDA) approved medications available for individuals with AD are called Cholinesterase Inhibitors. These medications help maintain levels of important chemicals in the brain, allowing the brain to function more effectively and slowing the progression of the disease. The four now approved medications are:

- Cognex (tacrine), not generally used due to side affects and is no longer actively marketed by the manufacturer

- Aricept (donepezil)

- Excelon (rivastigmine)

- Reminyl (galantamine)

Cognex was prescribed to my Mom … Her dosage was only half because of the side affects which may or may not have been effective. When she moved to Omaha and we met with Dr. Tim Malloy at the University Medical Center early in 1998, he prescribed the use of Aricept. Dr. Tim discussed with me about her current state, how there is no change in her memory. He also informed me of another new drug called Excelon, but said that it may or may not cause any noticeable changes since Mom's condition has greatly advanced. I agreed to try the drug, with a beginning dosage of 1.5 mg and increasing to 3 mg after two-three weeks. But after she had taken it a few weeks, it seemed to be making some changes in her to the extent that she responds to statements and also instructions. It was only a matter of months and we could no longer see any changes.

Different Stages of Alzheimer's Disease

Changes in the brain will bring about changes in the way the person reacts to his or her environment. These actions may seem out of character for the person. No matter how much they love you there is nothing they can do to stop the disease. AD begins slowly as it advances through the various stages.

Stage 1 (mild). It is said that this stage could last 2–4 years. During the days, weeks and months after moving back to Alabama began Mom's gradual memory lost. My Dad said that it began long before the moving, she just covered up a lot. We were just too preoccupied with our own issues of life to notice. I believe she realized something was wrong and began to pray more. The pressure of moving, all the uncertainty, not wanting to go, leaving her children and grandchildren behind, must have been hard.

Stage 2 (moderate). Ranges from 2–10 years. When we were in California in 1997, my sister and I knew that her condition was worsening. Every few minutes she was asking the same questions over and over … it was hard for us to digest the fact that maybe she didn't remember asking. She was constantly asking where Hick was—where was she and when are we going home.

When she returned to Omaha to live with me, she was in the short-term memory stage; always asking questions over and over (death of nerve cells in the brain). She had a genuine concern in her questioning. Perhaps she even thought we were ignoring her when we got tired of responding. This is where patience comes into play, as you will get tired of answering the same questions over and over again. We have to maintain that respect for our love one.

Towards the end of this stage, the individual begin having trouble translating thoughts into spoken words, and sometimes understanding, reading or writing. They become anxious, aggressive, or began to wander.

Stage 3 (severe). This stage can last 1–3 years or longer. Alzheimer patients can not do things on their own anymore. Can't use or understand words; can't recognize who they are in a mirror or family members. At this stage there is no return to reality, no return to being mom, knowing that here ends in death—the Alzheimer patient is usually institutionalized, which is the case with mom.

Final Stage. At this stage the individual is very vulnerable to infections of various types. Often unable to speak or communicate and the ability to walk is lost. There is urinary and fecal incontinence. Lost of the ability to swallow may cause choking and may lead to aspirations of food and secretions into the lungs, causing pneumonia.

Although Mom is still eating well, she sometimes experience problems with swallowing. But when it gets worse, we must now make sure that care is aimed toward reducing suffering and providing the best comfort and dignity. I know that when the time come, one day I will have to make a decision to use or not use feeding tubes and antibiotics.

Other Actions of Alzheimer's Patients

Social Engagement. There is a link between social engagement and cognitive performance. It has been proven that having social activities on a regular basis results in better cognitive performance. Evidence from studies of animals, nursing home residents, and community-dwelling of older people has suggested a link between social engagement and cognitive performance. Older adults who have a rich social network and participate in many social activities tend to have reduced cognitive decline and decreased risk of dementia.

The Friendship Program was a godsend. It offered social activities for Mom at a time when it was very much needed. Even if I had stayed home to care for her, it would not have been enough social activity to keep her active. Participating in this program helped her remain active and alert for over three years. I realized how important it was to keep Mom active and avoid isolation. I purposed to keep her surrounded with people who love her. My grandchildren helped me in this area.

Hiding and Losing Things. There were times mom would go into her room and close the door, rummaging through the drawers and closets. It didn't matter, because I felt she need her privacy and I wanted to make her as comfortable as possible. When she was in there for awhile, I would knock on the door and wait for a response. Then I would go in and sit on the bed, talking about anything and noticing how she had moved things around. There would be little items wrapped up in napkins in her drawer, under her pillow or in clothing that had pockets. Sometimes she would have taken everything out of the closet, including her suitcase trying to pack; other times she would have changed her clothes a couple of times.

Hallucinations, Illusions and Delusions. These mental aberrations are some of the most devastating symptoms of AD and are extremely difficult for caregivers to understand and accept. One way to address the problem, without causing undue concern, is to acknowledge the imagined article or situation and offer comfort to the individual.

I remember one particular evening, I was in the kitchen cooking and all of a sudden, Mom can running into the kitchen, excited and scared. I asked what was wrong and she responded in saying there was a man in the living room. I was a little concerned because during the summer months, I often left the front door open so she could venture out onto the porch, but the outside door was always locked. As we proceeded cautiously into the living room, it was a man on television who was in a threatening position. I was relieved and tried to get her to understand that it was just television. The best way I thought to handle the situation was to have her come into the kitchen and help with dinner.

Unexpected Actions. There were many incidents where I would have to take the mother role in our relationship. Mom loved to shop in her day, so I made it a point to take her to K-mart or Walgreen's when picking up her prescriptions. We even went to the shopping centers sometimes twice a week, just to get out of the house. Then she began to pick up items she did not need. Many times I had to discretely check her bag and/or pockets and if she had anything it usually was a small item and not costly. If it was something she did not need and was costly, I had to be creative in handling the situation.

There was an incident that I did not know how to handle while we were shopping in the J.C. Penney lingerie department. She did her usual walking around looking and then drifted over near the underwear. Before I could blink, she was at the counter taking money from her purse to pay for an item in her hand. After I had checked out, I asked her to put her money back into her purse and said that I had paid for it. She only had a few dollars and some change in her purse anyway. As she opened it, she pulled out a package of panties. I must admit I was not very tactful as I told her, "Mom, don't put things in your purse, they will put us in jail." Her response was that she didn't do that. This was offensive to both of us. She did an about face and started walking away. Immediately, I said come on lets go home—she dashed off down the escalator before me and waited at the bottom of the escalator. When I am angry, I get quiet and so does she so there was silence on the way home.

Driving. This activity involves multiple cognitive areas such as memory, orientation, spatial perception, reaction time and judgment. There is a time when driving can no longer be permitted. Although Mom had not driven since moving back to Omaha, she could tell you when a light is turning red or you are driving too close to the car in front of you.

One day Mom and I were going out and as we approached the car, she said she wanted to drive. I asked if she remembered how, since it had been a few years since she had driven, she answered yes. I said okay. She showed such excitement as she walked over to the driver's side … got in and waited until I got in. I was waiting outside because I didn't think she was serious. Praying as I got in, I handed her the keys. She put the key in the ignition, grabbed the steering wheel, looked forward and said, "I can't drive." She got out and came over to the passenger side. Never again did she ask or give any indication she wanted to drive.

Stubbornness and Uncooperativeness. Mom had to stop riding the Friendship van that picked her up each morning because they could not handle her. It was hard to get her on and off the van and due to the number of stops the driver had to make, it was impractical to continue picking her up. But there was a lady name Lillian who knew Mom prior to the Friendship Program, who took exception and put mom on her route, bringing her home sometimes in her own car. But she couldn't bring her home everyday. It was people like her who went beyond the call of duty and out of their way to make it easier for me.

Personal hygiene. Forgetting how much time has elapsed since the last change of clothing or taking a bath is common. Prior to one of my visits to Alabama, mom was changing often during the day, pulling clothes out of closet she had not worn in a while. But then she would come out with the same thing she had on the day before.

Wandering. Since most people with Alzheimer's disease wander, it is important to determine what is triggering the behavior. Wandering can be caused by a number of reasons and there's no way to predict when and how wandering might occur. My suggestion from experience is to be prepared.

There were many occasions that mom has wandered off, as mentioned in earlier chapters. It never failed, we would come home to relax before going back to the evening services and she would wait well until I was comfortable, then she'd get restless. The moment I closed my eyes she would move quietly and with such quickness towards the front door. I was beginning to believe she had some type of radar. There was one incident when I just let her walk out the door and I watched her go down the stairs and began walking up the sidewalk. I grab my keys and got in the car which was parked on the street. I followed her for some blocks thinking surely she would get tired. She crossed the streets cautiously and kept going straight. After she got to 16th Street, she turned and looked north towards my brother's house which must have been familiar to her. I got her attention and when she saw me, she stopped and got in the car.

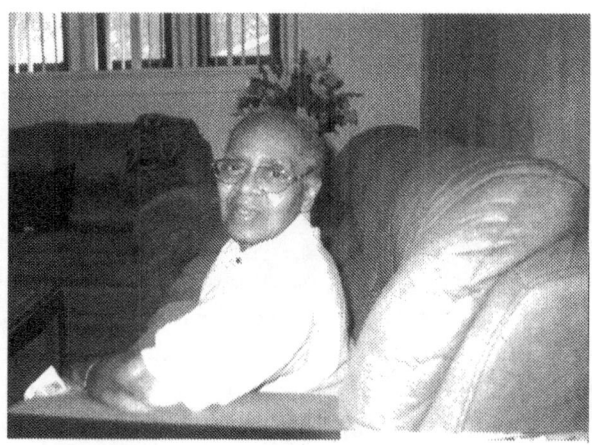

"A Sunday afternoon pose"

This evening action is called "sundowning." One in four Alzheimer patients become agitated in late afternoon or early evening which is a mysterious phenomenon. Some researchers think that these reactions maybe triggered by damage to the brain's sleep-wake rhythm.

Discussion During Doctor's Visit

On January 5, 2001, I took mom to Doctor Malloy's for her 3-month check up. Since her last visit in September, I was to reduce her Aricept dosage (10 mg) to every other day which I did, accept when she was in various nursing homes for respite. They won't change the dosage unless there is written documentation from doctor. When the nurse called her name, inquisitively and proudly she got up and followed her like nothing was wrong, she let the nurse take her temperature through the ear and she got upon the scale, then followed her to the examine room. She weighs 143 lbs, an increase of 3 lbs from four months ago; pressure sitting 134/70 and standing 122/74.

I had made note of some items I wanted to discuss with the doctor. Although he seems to have a genuine concern for his patients, I was feeling that he really doesn't check mom for other physical problems. I have to assume that her weight is ok; what about her pressure. Breast and pelvic, doesn't that matter anymore.

On this particular day he had asked her some usual questions like "what city do you live in, who are your parents, how many children you have and to name them.?" She didn't do very well although she tried, you could see the frustrations in her face, trying to remember. After Doctor Malloy had gone out, I asked her the same similar questions and she was able to answer them all. Now this is puzzling to me.

Mom takes *her partial* out a lot which cause me some concern. So I wanted to know if her gums are changing. He indicated that I should take her to the dentist. But that since she has lost weight and her mouth has reduced in size, it is understandable that her partial would be bothering her. I had tried to get her a dental appointment that same day at the medical center but it was a 3–4 month wait. I don't remember ever seeing my mom without her upper partial and most people didn't even know she had a partial. She and my Dad would always say that the dentist who made her partial, did a fantastic job in that it was a fit perfect. I remember when she had all her top teeth pulled, how she sort of stayed put until her partial was ready. She took it out only to clean and later on in life she'd let them soak over night.

There were several questions regarding her *sleeping habits*. There are times she will sleep 12–14 hours and I wanted to know if this is okay? His response was yes, and it will most likely increase as the disease progresses. It seems the more sleep she got, the less I got.

The plan was to take her back to Alabama again and I wanted to know what concerns he would have regarding *mom's travel?* I informed him that my last trip in 2000, I took her to Alabama and how well she did. He was concerned that the change would cause her to be irritable and whether I'd be able to handle her outburst. He indicated, if she was manageable then its okay. It didn't matter anyway, I was taking her. There needed to be some closure there.

Does she need flu shot? Yes, and so did I, indicating that it is too detrimental to not have one. Before we realize that we have the flu, the virus has already spread. He ordered a shot for her and wanted to give me one too, I had to decline since me and shots don't do well. Mom had her shot, and did well, but while on the table, she lost control of her bladder, which embarrassed her so and made her very irritable.

What does he consider the stage to consider permanent long term care? His reply was that I was far beyond this time. That was not what I wanted to hear, I had to disagree, and my level of care was not yet complete. I didn't feel God had released me, there was still more I was to learn about her, the disease and about myself, I felt I could go on further. The span of the disease on an average is about nine (9) years. Some at three years, some at twenty years, but the average is nine years from diagnosis. I indicated that it was about in 1996 that we first had her tested in Alabama.

What stage is my mom? He looked me in the eye and said "severe." It was like my thinking stopped there, because I was lost. Then he said on an average she has about 2-1/2 years remaining. Here I am a woman that believes in God and what he can do, and I am distraught over what this man is saying. My thought was how can he tell me how many years my mom has? The power of life and death lies in the hand of God, no man knows the hour or the day. It hurts so bad, even now as I write, anger rises in me, tears flow, because natural death is our destiny, separation from our loved one, but to live eternally with God, but being in the flesh, as we all are … we don't want to let go until we have no other choice.

Ending our visit, Dr. Malloy encouraged me to check into different facilities that would best meet my need since I work everyday and my job sometimes takes me out of town once a month. I need to make some unique scheduling and be flexible.

5

MY OWN PERSONAL STRUGGLES AS A CAREGIVER

o o o o o o o o o o o o o o o o o o o o o o o o o o o o o o o o o o
"Nobody knows the trouble I see, Nobody knows my fears; Nobody knows the road I travel, Nobody knows but me."

—*Unknown*

Caregiver is one who offers total care and support to individual(s) who are unable to function in a normal setting. They are faced with the mental, emotional, financial and physical challenges of providing 24-hour a day care as we painfully watch our loved one(s) slowly decline. Caregivers must assume new and unfamiliar roles in the family, most of which are both difficult and sad.

At some point in time, the question *"why me"* is probably asked by every caregiver. It was during various stages in my life, that I would ask God the same question and the answer is always the same, *"why not you."* I begin to think about what makes me so special that I should not be chosen for this task and I can come up with no answer.

As the baby boomers become of age, more and more of us are taking care of aging parents, as they are living longer and the cost of long term care is almost out of range, financially. Growing up I never envisioned caring for my parents; it was always assumed that we would all get old together. I never took time to think about what it would be like, or to think that far into the future. It was only after I got back from California in December 1997 that the care of my mother began taking first place in my thoughts.

After getting mom set up with a caseworker through the Social Security office and Health and Human Services, I was introduced to the Alzheimer's Associations Midlands Chapter. The initial call was made to Tia Scholfield and the conversation with her was a source of comfort to me. The only regret I have is that I didn't take advantage of all the services they offered.

I began to obtain information that was available and learn all I could about the disease and the affects it will have in the life of my mom. Although I felt alone, I constantly reminded myself that I was not. As I made various inquiries of friends and co-workers, I found out that many of them were in someway a caregiver for a parent or grandparent.

The experience of being a caregiver has taught me so much about life; how to appreciate and savor those special moments that so quickly fade away into distant memories. One thing is for certain, I believe God wanted me out of the "religious rat race" where you are constantly going and doing for others, never taking time for yourself or making yourself available to the voice of God. He had to slow me down and help me realize that it is He whom I should develop a personal relationship. Today I haven't gotten where I want to be, or where I should be but I am definitely not where I was a few years ago.

Resentment, Restoration, and Reason to Continue

For the first few months of this journey, I was holding unwarranted resentment in my heart. I resented my mother for allowing the disease to consume her; as if she had the power to resist. It is possible she fought as long as she could. I remember a conversation we had, she said that she waited but no one would come. I resented my father for not being there for her as she was falling deeper and deeper into the grasp of this disease. I resented my sister and brother for letting me take on the whole responsibility and seemingly not wanting to care for her as I do. I resented my children for not caring enough to go beyond their own issues of life. That all passed as I was maturing; realizing that God had chosen me to care for mom.

My care for Mom changed from obligation to "an honor." This is a "point of no return" in my life. I can no longer look at my mom and not see her as the "woman God's wants her to be." Now, as I bathe her, brush her teeth, comb her hair, dress her and sometimes feed her, it is for a queen who reigned well, a mother who gave birth to me, nurtured me, taught me the way of holiness, tended to my children, prayed for my broken marriage and accepted me for the decisions I had made up unto that point. Who could ask for anything else or better from a human being?

Providing care for an individual with dementia is one of the most difficult tasks imaginable, even more stressful than caring for a person with another illness.

People Are Placed in Our Lives for a Reason

I can identify with the author Mitch Albom in his book "Five People You Meet in Heaven." I do believe that God put people in your life for a reason and for a season. I had met Harrington Douglas in the summer of 1992 which would help shape my true understanding of being a caregiver. About a year after we met, he quit his job and moved back to St. Louis to care for his father who had been diagnosed with Alzheimer's disease. At first, he was ashamed to tell anyone of his father's condition, one who in the past was a vibrant retired postal worker. I had the opportunity to meet this elderly, energetic gentleman. As time progressed Harrington would share some of his daily experiences with me through phone calls, which came sometimes two and three times a day. I am reminded of the time he finally had to take his father's car keys and hide them. One day his dad had drove to the bank and came home without the car; and from then the slow progression of the disease. Harrington and I had not spoken in awhile, when one day he called in tears after he and his brothers decided to put their Dad into a nursing home. Guilt was overtaking him and he needed comfort in the decision they had made. His father died shortly after.

When he learned of my mother's diagnosis, he would encourage me to stay strong and gave me some helpful hints on handling certain issues that would surely arise. One thing that he said more than once and it stayed with me, "it won't be easy."

God Always Warns Us, If We Listen (August 8, 1998)

On last night Mom and I attend a revival at our church. A young lady from Barbados was praising God in the spirit of tongues. As plain as I speak, I heard the phrase, "fasten your seat belt." I've been wondering what this message meant, was it a warning for me or some accident coming or what—spiritually is my faith going to be tested?

I've been praying exceptionally hard this weekend because of the loneliness I have been experiencing and tiredness even though I've done hardly anything. To be honest, Mom is in a state of depression that also drains me. There is no laughter, no joy, just sadness and confusion and I am speaking of myself. She is more unsettled these days, but even through all this, she is as sweet as can be, just stubborn and want to be so independent. Definitely does not want to be corrected. She wants to be seen in the good which is natural.

It was the next week while on a work related trip to Reno, Nevada that I met Joe Bradley. He would bring lost love back into my life and change how I view a lot of things in life, especially love. This was so unexpected, and a romance of a lifetime.

Ready or Not, Changes Must Take Place

There were many changes in my own lifestyle that had to take place and I had to develop workable routines which made things go smoothly. I have always been somewhat flexible, but I had to become more comfortable with changes from day to day, learning to plan most aspects of my life to include my mom and her care. I needed to increase my knowledge in various skills to help me with the daily encounters.

There have been many embarrassing moments that have left me speechless, but I had to accept the fact that under normal circumstances, it would not have happened. I remember my friend Joe came to Omaha to visit for a few days. I took mom with me to the airport to pick him up, and then it was out to dinner with me and my guest. As we were eating, she took some of her food and wrapped it up in the napkin, which was a typical behavior I was use to. He asked if I knew what she was doing and I nodded as to agree, but rather than make a scene, which she has done in the past, I ignored it. As we are preparing to leave, I distracted her and took it away without her making notice of it.

You can not imagine the number of flatware she had brought home from the Friendship Program, wrapped up in a napkin. In fact, if there was anything she had to bring home it was wrapped up in a napkin or paper towel. I would clean them and return them at the end of the week.

She went everywhere with me, the doctor's, dentist, beauty shop; there was seldom a time when you saw me and she was not with me, with the exception of work. But, there were a couple of occasions where she did accompany me to work for an hour or two. Several aspects of my life changed for the better as our journey continued.

Humor is good for the heart. Laughing or giggling is part of my makeup, I find pleasure in laughing. It is said that laughter is good for the heart. Tensions are released, you breathe easier, the blood flows freely, and it is good. Mom would do and say things which brought about laughter, but since she can be very sensitive, I had to make sure that it was the appropriate time to laugh.

I remember we were having such a difficult time with our hair so I ordered wigs for both of us—she liked the "Tina Turner" hair style so I kept the other "curly cue," they both served its purpose. One day I said that we were wearing our hair to church and see what the reaction would be, she smiled and agreed. She wore "Tina Turner" and we did get a lot of response. When we got home, she and I laughed awhile at the stares and the imagined comments.

On another occasion after a long day, I had made sure Mom was nice and comfortable in bed. After I finished a few chores, I had gotten into bed and was almost ready to fall off to sleep. I turned and there standing in the door way was Mom, fully dressed, along with hat and coat. I had to hold back the laughter and just say "Eula Mae where are you going." It was always the same answer, "I'm going home." My quiet response would be, "Oh God" then I would then get up and get her back into bed.

In dealing with various problems, there are times you need to step back from it and think on something else. That's when I would remember one of the conversations with my friend, Joe Bradley. He had a great sense of humor, and was able to push my funny button—he had this thing about Omaha and cows. I don't know if I believed him or not but he said that he had never met any one of color from Nebraska and thought that this was just a small country town with lots of cattle roaming the streets. I would think of some hilarious comment he made and break out into a laugh and it always made me feel better.

Pray for patience. There were times I was so tired that if she did get up out of the bed, I wouldn't move but listen as she tries to walk quietly down the stairs in the dark. The moment it got too quiet, I was up and down the stairs. Sometimes she'd be sitting on the sofa, other times she'd be in the kitchen or just going from room to room. I never had a problem with her wandering out the front door at night because the stairs made squeaking noise when you walked down, and believe me there were plenty of stairs. Also, the front door had an alarm that sound when opened.

Keeping Balanced. I never really gained total balance in my life but I tried. Many times I failed but never giving up. There is an old hymn titled "I found the answer, I learned to pray" which became the key to what balance I had. Being a grandmother, mother, sister, and daughter of a person with Alzheimer's can be difficult. I even tried to prioritize my life to include my job which I enjoyed. My director, Don Lightwine, played an important role in my getting my act together at work. Much of the pressure was relieved through his taking the time and having the concern to sit down with me and talk about my situation. I remember at lease two occasions going into his office, opening up, crying and sharing some of my frustrations. He always made me feel that he had a genuine concern for my well being and my success on the job. Working in a large corporation as this, personal concerns for the employees is not top priority. I will be ever grateful for the opportunities he afforded me.

Needing Emotional Support. I believe if it was not for the support of my family and pastor, I could not have made it this far and in return I was able to be there for my mom. There were many times she tried to express herself but it was as if something is blocking her thought process and not allowing her to complete what she began to say. I tried to understand and be there when she wanted to talk and regularly reassured her that it was okay to talk about anything, and that it was okay if she didn't get the correct words in the right place.

When Overwhelmed, Ask for Help (February 15, 1998)

Ask family members and friends to spend time with the individual so you can attend to other important matters or just take a break to shop or have alone time. It has always been difficult for me to ask for help, even from my own family. But I finally broke down and asked my brother, my mother's only son for help with mom. He came over late as usual on Sunday evening just as we were about to go back to church evening services. As we sat and looked at television, I prayed that God will give me the words and the courage to speak with him. I don't know what's so hard about asking a son for help with his mother. I explained her situation and also gave him a couple of books on the subject Alzheimer's disease. My purpose was for him to be able to recognize some of her symptoms and what to expect. My brother is a quiet nature man which is one of the traits of the Samuel family, so he never really said a lot, just listened to what I had to say and then said he'd do whatever I wanted him to do. As much as I love my only brother, even that didn't sound good enough for me.

I guess I was looking for him to take control of the whole situation. I don't want to feel like "Teen it's your show." I'm expecting too much I know and I am going to try real hard to cope with these feelings I have. My dad was always proud to say that his sister, Aunt Alice took care of his mother in her days of ailment and later demise; how he sent her money to help in her care. That was good but there can never be enough money to pay for this type of care.

Life is funny in that we live it without really understanding it. God is sovereign and he knows all about us—it is hard for us to understand his plan for us.

Sometimes I just shut out my thoughts because it's all in vain. Its like why even ask when you know it is probably not in the plan—the scripture Isaiah 55:8 says, *"For my thoughts are not your thoughts ... "* so why waste the time and energy.

April 8, 2000

The Sizzler Restaurant was one of our favorite hangouts for dinner on Saturday or Sunday. Sitting here I notice how observant I have become of older people and how they interact with each other. As Mom and I sat eating our dinner, I watched all the elderly folks and one couple caught my attention. They were very short in statue and maybe of orient decent. They went through the buffet line slowly, deciding what to put on their plates. The gentlemen assisted the woman as they got their food and went to their seats. He returned to the food counter and she watched him without distraction, all the way there and back. When he returned to his seat, she began to eat. Out of all the couples I had seen there, they were the only ones talking to each other. I began to wonder to myself how long they had been together or even if they were married. Were there any children? It is times like this that reinforce my desire to have someone to grow old with, to hold my hand as I drift away into that eternal sleep.

Wow, is this me talking like this? Yes it is, the older we get we realize that life as we know it, is not forever. But the love we share continues beyond.

January 27, 2001

After dinner, Mom and I sat down and watched a movie on television called "My Sister's Keeper." It was at a time in my life when I struggle within myself. The story was of how a retarded daughter remained in care of the mother, while the other daughter went off to become an acclaimed artist. The successful daughter seemed ashamed of her home situation. After the mother died, she toiled with the decision to continue the care of her sister. It concluded with the realization that she is "her sister's keeper." Many of the scenes reminded me of mom's care, how there were times when we would be out and I'd be so embarrassed by the way she responded to me.

This time last year our morning struggles really began and yet I look back and wonder if I could have handled various situations better; maybe so if I had experience the situation before. I tried for three years and six months—it doesn't seem that long ago that this journey began Christmas 1997. The progression of the disease isn't moving fast and that's good it allows me more time to adjust. Most times she can't form her words but there are times we can understand what she is saying.

We have to learn to cope with the stress associated with care giving. And, we never stop hearing the instructions of "take care of your self." I don't know if I learned to cope with the stress associated with care giving but I do acknowledge that it is my faith and trust in God that helped sustain me. Yes, I neglected myself many times but my family and friends were a great source of support, which did allow me to take breaks.

Love makes us think that we can do and accomplish anything and if given an opportunity again, I would do it again but with more knowledge of the disease. It is impossible to imagine the enormous demands on the caregiver. The AD affects every family member, making deep permanent changes. You don't think about how you will replenish your supply of patience, tact, humor and maintain a sense of balance.

6

COPING WITH MY DECISION: THE DAYS, MONTHS AND YEARS THAT FOLLOW.

"Coping with the Seasons of Life—it is just a season. Some observations can only be made by living, and knowing how to adjust to your situation."

—*Quote from 2006 sermon delivered by*
Bishop Scott of Southern Illinois Jurisdiction

For weeks I had toiled with the thought of making a decision to have mom moved to a nursing facility and I know the decision must come soon. I just want someone to tell me "okay now is the time, let's do it now." But no, this is someone's life, even if this was told to me I wouldn't accept it. Mom and I never talked about this; I don't know what her wishes would be other than she was a very independent woman, and it would be the last resort before she would ask for help. I never want to put my children through this, at least not one alone. I want to be in a position that when I get old and can't get around, my children will know what my desires are. I will make it known.

I made an appointment with a nice young attorney who was a friend of my daughter. Before going, I asked Mom if she wanted me to take care of her money business and medical business and she said yes. I told her what we were going to do and although somewhat puzzled, she agreed. The attorney made her feel comfortable and not on the defensive. After the documents for power of attorney were prepared, she again agreed and signed the necessary papers.

March 1, 2001

The time of decision has finally come. I've avoided the thought of this day for a long time. I am going to take her to the nursing home and in doing so I will have to put her on several waiting lists. It is confusing how Medicare works so there were many calls to mom's caseworker. According to Medicare, she must be hospitalized before entering into the nursing home, before they would pay for long term care; and, Medicaid has a different set of stipulations.

Nursing homes are quite expensive, more than a monthly mortgage payment, but I can understand why. Just with the expense of caring for my mom, time has a high value. Many of the workers at the nursing homes have families, their own homes and their own time; even with that they can say enough is enough. But when you are a caregiver, it goes far beyond that. We just can't say I'm not doing this today, although I felt like it many times.

April 24, 2001

This morning before coming downstairs I hugged Mom and told her I loved her so very much; the tears just rolling. Does she know what is going on with me? Does she realize the stress I am under, toiling with the decision that must be made? How can I tell a woman, still full of laughter although at times so sad, that I can no longer care for her?

When I am dressing her, it feels like someone dressing me … when I lotion her legs; rub her back, it feels like someone is doing that for me. I guest the point that God is trying to get across to me is "do for her the way you want someone to do for you."

I hug my grandchildren whenever they come into my presence and sometimes maybe too much. Now and then I ask my sons, daughter and even son-in-law to hug me. My pastor always say, there are people who have not been hugged in a long time, and that is so true being single, it gets lonely at times, sometimes going days without a human touch. When someone does embrace you, you don't want to let go, my inner thoughts are "hold me a little longer please." And I try to do that with mom; shower her with hugs and kisses.

Bathing her has become easier and I no longer have to struggle with her, not because she is weaker but because I am changing. I look at her often with her countenance so sad, then she will catch my eye; and sometimes smile and then there are times she gets defensive.

I would leave a light on in the bathroom, so she could easily see where it was. Her consistency at night was becoming more of a problem. There were times that she would have a bowel movement at night, so in the morning there was clean up tasks. It was puzzling to me how she would hide it in a shoe box or a shoe, under her pillow, under the bed. As that stage changed and believe me I was glad, I had to start just cleaning her up.... I finally have learned to use the rubber gloves. In sharing this information with my sister, Liz and I began praying that she would get back onto schedule. I don't want her to be constipated, but regular during the day. Now she moves around and gets up walks.

Final Decision Is Made

Well, I finally made the decision regarding mom's long term care. It's set, on June 23, 2001 at 11:00 AM she will become a resident of Maple Crest Nursing Home. In my discussion with the facility, I will be picking her up on the weekends, Saturday and Sundays and sometimes on Friday evening. This decision has been a long time coming and I am still uneasy about taking her. I know that God is giving me the strength to do what must be done.

I have had butterflies in my stomach, even diarrhea.... it's like something else is about to happen. I have been praying for guidance ... wishing someone would make the decision for me, telling me it's not the right thing to do, tell me something.... When I share my plan with people, they say "Well you are blessed to have been able to care for her this long" or you have done as much as you can, etc. But no one says "hang in there, try a little longer. I even get upset when someone sounds disappointed that I am giving up. Am I giving up ... really am I?

I constantly think about Aunt Mary, my mom's youngest sister. How she cared for Big Mama (my grandmother) for years until her death ... I try to figure out why I can't follow pursuit. Mary had a little more support than I as she didn't work outside the home at the time, she had children at home who could help, a husband for support; all of which I do not have. As most, I am always trying to justify my actions. Would it have been better if I had a husband to support me at a time like this? Only the Lord knows. No sense tossing that around.

Another New Home (June 23, 2001)

Saturday morning, I got her up which was quite easy, dressing her carefully. I was able to shampoo and curl her hair without any problems. As I was finishing up, I fell on my knees before her, looked into her eyes, and she into mine. As tears began to roll down my cheeks, I laid my head in her lap as a confused child longing for the touch of that caring mother. She put her arms around me and began to rock, it was for just a brief moment but it felt so good. It was at that time I realized she knew me and the test I was going through.

The night before, my daughter and I worked on her room, putting up pictures, adding plants, a rug and some of her things from my house. We did everything to make the room as comfortable as possible. I couldn't help remembering all the times she made us feel so comfortable in her home. My daughter said it reminds her of a dorm room.

Mom went to the nursing home without any problems, as many times before. After getting her all settled in, I stayed until lunch time. As I began to leave she followed me to the door, showing me in all her expressions that she wanted to go also. The nurse aid kindly distracted her while I went out the door. Leaving her at the nursing home was harder for me than for her. I felt as though I was abandoning her, letting her down. I felt like a failure and wanted to try again. I find myself alone again battling within the fact that this was the right decision and the right time.

June 24, 2001

During the orientation prior to her becoming a resident, they had informed me that there would be an adjustment period needed. All they were saying was that I should allow her time to adjust and not visit much. I was up, showered and at the nursing home about 7:00 AM. It had been hard for me to sleep last night knowing that she was there and not home with me.

It was lonely already at the house. It was the same at church, without her at my side. However, I was encouraged through the testimonies and the word of God brought forth. I Stopped at Target to pick up birthday cards and came home. Such a lonely afternoon, just knowing she was not here. I was on my way back out to visit her around 4:30 PM.

June 30, 2001

Everyday, I would find myself there at the home visiting in the evenings during workdays and mornings and noon on weekends. When I did get home it seems I am more exhausted than if she was there with me.

July 1, 2001

I attended the Samuel family reunion held in Pensacola, Florida—this is the first time I had come home and mom was not there—it seemed so strange to be in Mom and Dad's house without her. It was the first reunion I've attended without her around, but I tried to make up for it when I returned to Omaha. She seems to be adjusting well to her new home. I now pick her up on Saturday mornings and return her on Sunday evenings. She still enjoys the church services and still likes to be on the go. I am finding it difficult to get her in and out of the car. I guest if I were comfortable; I wouldn't want to move either.

Feeling Lost (July 20, 2001)

What will I do today? I am constantly trying to fill my time with something else to do. It has been 3 ½ years of caring for Mom night and day. Since placing mom in the nursing home, I am almost lost. These feelings of being lost, whether in direction or in life in general, it is not good, it is devastating. I don't see how I could have cared for her as I did, but I still have the memories and the good still out weighs the bad. I look forward to seeing her in the evenings and picking her up on Saturday mornings, keeping her until Sunday evening. She remembers me … One day she even told the nurse the names of the persons on the pictures in her room, even that dad was her husband.

The following weeks were very tiresome, almost a strain. All I want to do now is sleep, I don't cry much, don't pray much, don't go to church much, nothing much. It's almost like I just exist, waiting on a change. I wonder if this is what Mom was talking about when she said "she tried to wait, but no one would come." Waiting on what, I don't know and who. Being a woman of faith, it must have been a stage in her life where she was waiting on deliverance from God. Then did she just give up? Being isolated, as she was, perhaps there was no one to help pray her through … did she cry out and received no answer?

September 1, 2001

Mom seem distant today, she was not laughing, seemed awfully tired—took her to the Dairy Queen for her favorite strawberry sundae. This has been one of our Sunday afternoon rituals when we don't go to the Sizzler Restaurant down the street. We returned to the home and I put her to bed.

Shopping Day

I picked Mom up on Friday after work. She was spending the night. She was always excited when she knew she was going out. She would stand close to me while I checked her out for two days, as if for some reason they wouldn't let her go. We got up early, ate breakfast and were out the door before 10:00 AM. She was so excited about going anywhere. Arriving back at the house, we enjoyed a relaxing evening watching television. In fact our weekend consisted of going to church, out to dinner and visiting a few folks.

While shopping at the famous Wally World (Wal-Mart), I let her push the cart up and down the isles, picking up some small items. At times, she would stop and pick up an item and stare at it; possibly remembering something about it. By the time we got to the check out, I had put back most of the items we didn't need. But I was not going to take the pleasure of filling the cart from her. She even wanted to push the cart to the car. It was a good day for her.

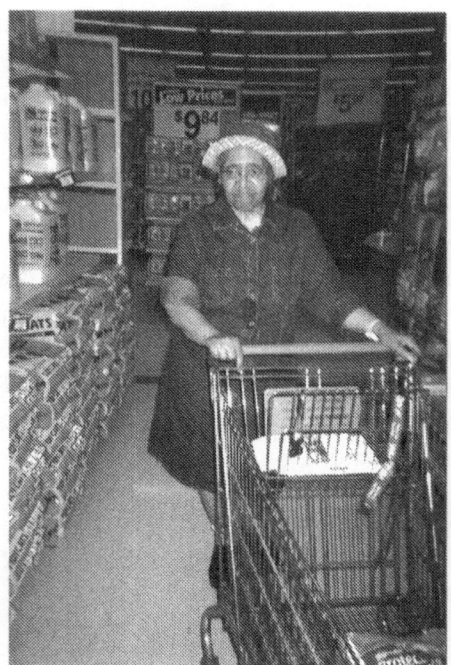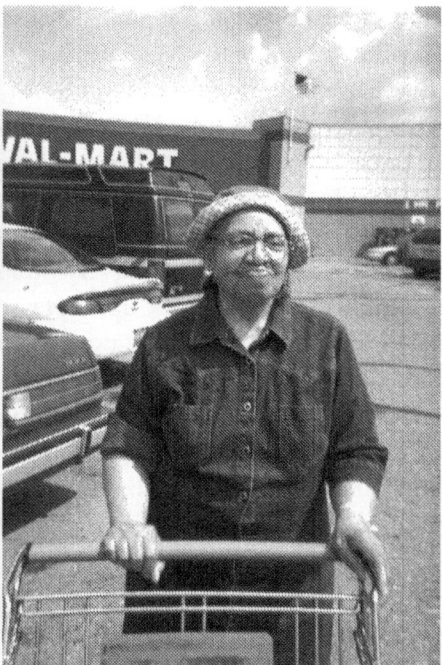

Shopping at Walmart

September 6, 2001

Mom was in a very upbeat mood as I visited with her. While there, we called Dad on the phone and they talked, with her looking over at me smiling and saying a few words.

November 2, 2001

Mom is adjusting well at the nursing home—I try to visit daily and when she see me, that familiar expression comes over her face, so surprised and glad to see me. I want her to be as happy as she can be—she still acknowledges prayer and participates. I'm slow in that area and need to pray more with her.

Happy Birthday (December 26, 2001)

Mom spent Christmas with me, which we both thoroughly enjoyed. When it was bedtime, she slept with me because I didn't feel comfortable leaving her in the room alone. It was such a treat for the both of us and it was like she had never left—she does not move at all, sleeps real still. I got close to her and made myself comfortable; me the little girl, she my mom. I then remember how it feels to be lonesome, longing for the touch of a human hand, so I rubbed her forehead and placed my hand on her shoulder, she smile. She didn't get too irritable, until Christmas day. It was because I was overbearing in my authority, I told her to come on, when we were leaving Hope's house, then I snapped my finger, that set her off. I guess if it were me, I would have felt the same way.

Today we are having cake and ice cream for mom at the nursing home. She is 72 today. God is good. I can't believe that I have not written much this year … so much has happened since the beginning of the year but I could not have been that busy.

January 5, 2002

My cousin Ronnie brought Aunt Ruby, mom's sister, up from Kansas City for a short visit with mom. The look on mom's face when she saw Aunt Ruby is to be remembered and cherished. She knew exactly who she was. They talked, laughed and cried the entire visit.

February 17, 2002

Growing up, each morning if we came downstairs for breakfast exceptionally early, we would find mom at the kitchen table, hands grasped together in prayer. Breakfast was always prepared and ready to eat. Those prayers morning after morning, she was sending up her timber. When I remember those mornings, it reminds me of the role I now play in her life. How her care changed from duty and obligation to "honor."

March 27, 2002

I really want to finish my manuscript but I just can't find the time to write. Mom is doing well, in fact better than what the doctors predicted a year ago. Even though she is in the nursing home, I worry about her being in an atmosphere that is stable. She remains on the medication Excelon, Procardia for her pressure and Depakote to keep her emotions under control.

I was so tired when I visited her yesterday evening. I laid my head back as I sat in her chair and dosed off—I was awaken by something she was mumbling, then when I made eye contact she asked "you sleep?" She was looking straight at me, like I look at her when she sleeps. She still has the concern of a loving mother but she can no longer form the appropriate words. When she recognizes someone her facial expressions show it, through her enlarged eyes and her raised cheek bones.

She has gained most of her weight back, now in a size 20 now. When her garments are too short, she still pulls it down over the knees; she has beautiful legs. I can see the difference in me each day I go out to visit her. I'm so glad to see her—I know what it feels like to be lonely. It is a true statement that people forget about you when you are out of their presence. That's why not many days go bye without my seeing her; I don't want her to forget me and I want to be there when she remembers, if for only a moment. Others, well everyone has their own lives and concerns and it is not their responsibility.

Mom is getting pretty good care here at Maple Crest but I am also trying to do my part—I keep doing her laundry as a sort of connection, plus I keep tabs on her clothes and what she wears. I give firm instructions to the aides that at all times she is fully dressed for her meals. That means all her undergarments, including stockings or socks. I give her a pedicure and manicure at lease twice a month. She has always had corns on her outer toes, one of the many traits I inherited from her. It is important for me to keep up her appearance, because if and when she ever wakes up and say "I am back" like my dream in 1997; then she would be proud of how I cared for her.

April 2, 2002

Here it is months later, and I have not been keeping up on my notes. Mom is doing well at the home and she still remembers me. And to our surprise she remembers others and at times is able to communicate. When I mention those Samuel hips, she smiles … all her skirts are too small … the weight has slowed her down somewhat. The caregivers at the nursing facility take good care of her which is a blessing. I am there in the evenings and sometimes drop in during the day, which makes a difference in the care she receives. We have her on a schedule. We went to church this past Easter Sunday and she seems to enjoy it, and she still likes music. I try to get her to sing more but she basically hums the tune to the songs.

A few weeks ago, Aunt Ruby came up from Kansas City where she is now living. I have just learned that she has the beginning stages of Alzheimer's disease and is on medication. How can this be, another great woman of God.

April 24, 2002

She remembers me and she responds to "mama." If you stare at her she'll say "what" and smiles. She will be coming home for a few days around mother's day—my sister will be here.

I want to try again to take mom to Alabama. If only I could get someone to go with me. I am curious to know how she will react. She answers when I call her "mom."

At the home in the Alzheimer's unit, they had an artist come in and paint the locked doors from the inside. The scenes are beautiful; there is a fence and then lots of flowers. This is to distract the residents from trying to go out the door, as they often did.

May 13, 2002

This was a great Mother's Day weekend; it was my brother's birthday and my eldest son's birthday. Mom came home with us Saturday and spent the night with me and my sister who is home for a few days. Everything went well with her enjoying the time with us and we definitely enjoyed her.

June 24, 2002

After dinner, mom and I did our little power walk up and down the halls. As we walked, I filled her in on the family news at home. A few weeks ago when we first started, we went around the entire building once. I noticed that she was so red but she didn't seem tired. I asked the nurse to take her pressure and she was fine. That's all I wanted to hear, so I said "let's go" and we did a second round. But today I felt led to pray—at the end of the prayer we began to sing, ending in one of our favorite hymns "Yes Lord." Tears began to build up in her eyes. Although it was just a few moments, she was aware of the power of praise and prayer. I thought to myself, it's still there. I'll never know when it will be my last time speaking to her, hearing her laugh and sometimes get a few words out. But each time I touch her, rub her shoulders, massage her hands, I am, with all my heart doing unto her as I would have someone do unto me.

July 13, 2002

Today I picked mom up for the weekend. When we arrived at the house, she just looked around as if the place was new to her; then she looked over at me. I wonder what is going through her mind, has she forgotten the place she lived for three years? Things have changed in the past two years. On Sunday we got dressed and off to church without any problems. She had even fed herself at breakfast and ate quite well.

February 9, 2003

At Maple Crest, mom's area is called Maple Terrace, which is the Alzheimer's unit. Mom is sitting quietly as she feeds herself and makes sure she sees everyone who enters the dining room. It takes her awhile, sometimes up to an hour; she chews slowly as she looks around. She is alert and smiles at the laughter around her or when someone says something funny.

April 30, 2003

Sitting here watching her eat dinner, I am remembering back five years ago this past Good Friday, how mom walked away from the Friendship Program (Adult Day Care). She is still able to feed herself with some preparation of her foods. She does not talk much any more, there are times I think she forgets she don't talk and will say a few words, and then it's hard to understand what she is saying. It's not my imagination, she still remembers me. Some may say that it's an assumption since I desperately want her to talk to me. She doesn't walk much, especially alone. My brother and I, when visiting make sure we walk her up and down the halls. But with the lack of exercise and her additional weight, she has to be motivated to walk. But when she does, she still has that strut, and that pleasant smile when she meets someone in passing.

Nursing homes are struggling to keep good employees on the salaries they pay. So, there is always someone new to get to know. There are fewer volunteers, and less visits by family members. I can understand why she is not walked on a regular basis, they lack help.

May 15, 2003

My visits to the nursing home are almost daily and I try to vary my times on weekends. Saturdays I get there at breakfast but most times I try to be there at lunch and dinner on Sunday. The rest of the week it is at dinner unless I am off work.

Today was a little stressful, I felt tensed and don't know the reason. I could sense tension as I was feeding mom. She wasn't eating fast enough and she wouldn't get up out of the chair. I tried to help her up but it was like dead weight to lift her but she does not help any; when lifting her feet while she is sitting is like lifting a large number of pounds. I found myself getting angry at her for not trying. One thing I will not tolerate is my forcing her to do anything, and getting angry about it. As I prepared to leave, I told her I needed to stay away a few days, gave her a kiss and left.

Can't she see my devotion,
all my effort in trying to keep her active, alert and mobile?
Why won't she cooperate with me?

I refuse to accept the diagnosis that she may never walk alone again; never carry on a conversation; never be the mother I so desperately need at times.

May 16, 2003

When you have mobility, other body functions work—when Mom walks, her head moves, her eyes have movement, she is turning looking into rooms, at other individuals in passing; yes, her hands shake but she is reacting. When she is in the wheelchair, she is just a not on a log.

June 28, 2003

Dad has been here since Friday of last week. It was a busy day today but we took time to visit mom about 7:00 P.M. which was a little later than usual. They had already put her in bed but she was not asleep, so Dad and I just sat beside her bed and watched TV. Amazingly, Mom edged up on her arms and after a few minutes, she sat up all alone for about 10 minutes. In our amazement, she started smiling, I think she surprised herself. We just started laughing with joy. This was great to see her set up on her own ability, since before now; she had not been sitting up without assistance.

June 29, 2003

Tonight, in preparing Mom for bed, I had taken her to the shower room and had one of the assistants to help me get her out of the wheelchair onto the toilet. I thanked the assistant and as she was leaving, low and behold mom said "thank you" to her also. Again, this is surprising since she does not talk anymore. If she does, her words are not understandable.

August 19, 2003

Watching her tonight, my mind goes back to how things have changed. Her smiles are not as frequent, her response to "mom" is sporadic; they don't even walk her anymore, if anything it is due to her weight and degenerative knee. She has always had problems with her left knee. I had been walking her from the shower room and each time she would liven up; the blood get to flowing and the smiles came. I haven't walked her in awhile. She stares a lot with lack of interest, yet this lady retains her integrity. She lets you know in her expressions when her body is exposed or when someone strange touches her.

August 28, 2003

When people found out where she was, they would say things like "you are a good daughter, you did your best, God's going to bless you for caring for your mom as long as you did; or it was time." Nothing they said made me feel any better or remove the pain I was feeling. "God has a blessing for you, a reward stored up in heaven for your dedication to your mother." I would trade that blessing any day just to have her back as "Mom."

March 14, 2004

Mom's state is somewhere between stages 3 and 4, she doesn't talk but she does respond with "yes." She yet hums familiar tunes ... she still holds proper items in her hands and while eating she puts food in her mouth and chews slowly, even without any teeth. She still does things when she feel no one is looking, like pick up a spoon or cup; she will only look at you when you are not looking her way, when eye contact is made she looks away.

November 14, 2004

Mother was very active today, she said a few words of which I could not understand and she was humming. I had the doctor take a look at her mouth; it seems that the abscess on her gums is getting larger. He indicated that to have her teeth removed may cause complications, with her being under anesthesia. He suggested that we keep them clean and on antibiotics for any infections. That just doesn't sound right me.

Sometimes we relinquish our concerns to the Doctor's prognosis. That is wrong. As a caregiver one must weigh all the options. You know the patient sometimes better than anyone, knowing when they are in pain or when something else is wrong. I accepted the doctor's suggestion on the issue of removal of her teeth long enough. I then demanded that they remove them. Although she could not tell us she was in pain, I had to reach back and remember when I had bad tooth aches, then imagine her pain was much more. The oral surgery went well and after removal of all her remaining teeth, she did so much better.

January 1, 2005

Another year has past, and we are all still here. Mrs. Eula Mae has surpassed the time predicted by doctors.

February 18, 2005

Mom seems to be having problems swallowing today. As I am feeding her, I massage her throat and sort of help with the mouth movement. Her eyes look exceptionally weak, especially the left eye, red around the lids. Yet after dinner sitting with her, she seems alert, looking around; staring at me when I am not looking. When I asked her a question, she looks at me as if she is trying to understand. She holds my hand with a tight grip giving some movement … she smiles at some commercials on the TV that catches her attention.

I am writing fewer lines as I gradually get back into a life of being a parent and grandparent.

October 29, 2005

Some of the grandchildren were out visiting Mom today at lunch. Nolen and the twins were so excited about feeding "Granny." They love to say "open Granny" and she would open wide, afterwards they'd say "good job Granny." I wonder will they care for me when I am old?

7

NOW UNTIL THEN: ONLY GOD KNOWS WHEN

o o o o o o o o o o o o o o o o o o o o o o o o o o o o o o o o o o

"The strongest and sweetest songs yet remain to be sung."

—*Walt Whitman*

Life is the existence of changes as nothing remains the same. It is the words of Solomon in the book of Ecclesiastes, where he speaks of the appropriate seasons of life. This reveals facts that help deal with the "menu" of life.

> *"To ever thing there is a season, and a time to every purpose under the heaven. A time to be born, and a time to die; a time to plant and a time to pluck up that which is planted. A time to kill, and a time to heal; a time to break down and a time to build up; a time to weep, and a time to laugh; a time to mourn, and a time to dance. A time to cast away stones and a time to gather stones together; a time to embrace, and a time to refrain from embracing; A time to get, and a time to lose; a time to keep and a time to cast away; A time to rend and a time to sew; a time to keep silence, and a time to speak; A time to love and a time to hate; a time of war and a time of peace."*

> —*Ecclesiastes 3:1–8*

Today, I look back and wonder how and why all of these changes take place in our lives and come to the realization that since there is a beginning, there is an end. In between is a process that must take place in order to complete the cycle; whether it is a project your working on or even the inevitable, death.

In my closing, I'd like to share this letter composed in 2001; but never sent to my family because I never found the appropriate time.

Well, loved ones,

It is getting closer to the time of a most crucial decision that I will have to make, which will affect all our lives. I have been caring for my mom, your wife, mother, grandma, aunt, and sister since December 1997. What started as a "duty" turned into an "honor".

She is getting to the point that my care is not sufficient enough, where her human dignity is not diminished in anyway. Mom is a great lady; she was devoted to her husband, she loves God, her children and grandchildren. She was and is a very independent woman, which has its advantages and disadvantages in life.

This disease has stripped her of so many things, it's hard to explain. Watching her change by the day sometimes is unbearable for me, but God strengthens me for the next day. In November 1999, I began to take her to the nursing home for respite while I was out of town for whatever reason. The first time was the most difficult because I felt that I was deserting her, shying away from my responsibility for selfish reasons. Driving to the airport I wanted to turn around, go back and pick her up to resume my care of her. It was only because of my job that I did not do it.

Each time I think of this time of decision, tears form and I tell myself that God will help me make the right decision at the right time.

I talked to Aunt Mary and admonished her for her care of her mom and Aunt Hattie Mae. As most of you, I had no idea of the burden or task in caring for an elderly person, especially one with Alzheimer's disease.

My reason for writing is twofold; it is a release for me, all the notes, the late night prayers, restless sleep and the need for you to know about this lady from my perspective; about this disease and how it destroys life as we know it.

I have been praying that God will heal this condition; praying asking why? I never knew Mom to intentionally hurt anyone, not even my Dad. I have learned so much about her that I never knew or understood, I even see a lot of myself in her, only she suppressed a lot of her feelings, a lot of anger was held inside.

Before she was unable to communicate, she shared a lot of things with me and I then began to ask her questions, some she could answer, at least she wanted to. She loved my dad, but I'll never understand that obsessive feeling she had for him. Perhaps I shall never experience the true love shared by my forefathers and mothers. Although it seems as though she was starved for attention, in return she has always been a caring and affectionate person—I don't know if that is something that came in later years or was always there.

My mentality is still good, but I know that if I continue to struggle trying to balance my life to include her care, care of myself, being a mother and grandmother, there is a point of no return and I am almost there.

I love my job and don't plan to quit, God be willing I want to retire.

> *Sincerely,*
> *Your mother,*
> *Grandmother,*
> *Daughter,*
> *Sister,*
> *Niece,*
> *Cousin,*
> *and Friend.*

Now Until Then

Day after day I visit the nursing home, smiling and calling her name; massaging her head, arms and back, and feeding her. Sitting with her, hearing her hum an unknown tune while watching our favorite game show, Wheel of Fortune, I am hoping to capture the moment when she remembers and calls my name—I am longing to hear her once again give verbal praise to God. Many times I call out to her, "Mom, Mom, Mama, let me know your still there." She just looks at me and at times smiles. That will have to do until tomorrow.

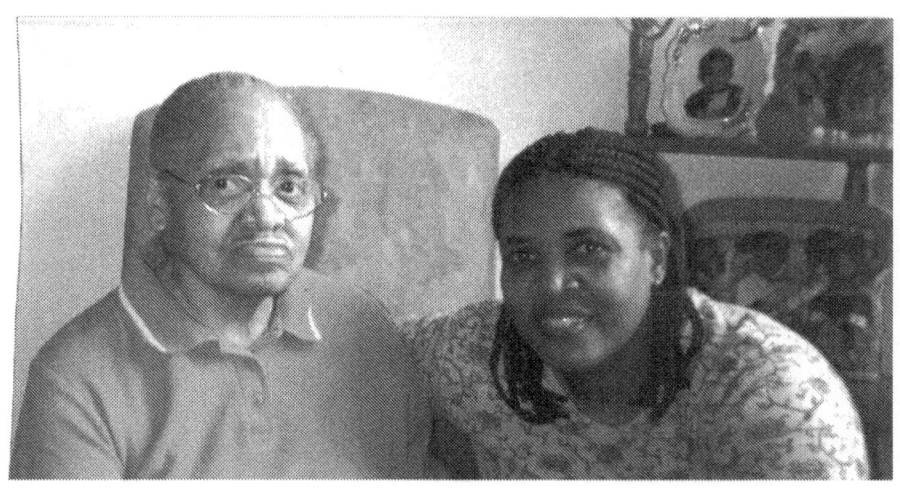

Eula and Teen

Unless I should die tonight, tomorrow I will visit her again and again until then.

"She doesn't sing anymore
but one day on the other side of the far shore,
that known thief will have to return what was taken,
and the song on her lips and in her heart, God will restore."

Ernestine

RESOURCES

Alzheimer's Disease Publications Catalog
Contact:
Alzheimer's Disease Education and Referral (ADEAR) Center
P O Box 8250
Silver Spring, MD 20907-8250
E-mail: adear@alzheimers.org
Website address: http://www.alzheimers.org

Trading Memories: An Adolescent's Guide to Alzheimer's Disease, 1997
American Health Assistance Foundation
15825 Shady Grove Road, Suite 140
Rockville, Maryland 20850
Website address: http://www.ahaf.org

Simpson, Robert and Anne. Through the Wilderness of Alzheimer's: A guide in Two Voices
1999 Augsburg Fortress

Living With Alzheimer's Disease: A Guide for Caregivers, 1998 Pfizer Inc and Eisai Inc.
An educational program sponsored by Pfizer Inc and Eisai Inc.

Caregiver Guide
U.S. Dept of Health and Human Services, Public Health Service
National Institutes of Health, National Institutes on Aging
2004

Alzheimer's Disease: Unraveling the Mystery, 2004
National Institute on Aging, National Institutes of Health

Alzheimer's Disease Fact Sheet
U.S. National Institues of Health, National Institute on Aging
http://www.nia.nih.gov/Alzheimers/Publications

What is Alzheimer Disease?
www.alzheimer.ca

Alzheimer's Association, Midlands Chapter Newsletter
www.midlandsalz.org

Alzheimer's Disease: Assessment, Diagnosis and Treatment
Center for Aging, Alzheimer's Disease & Neuro-degenerative Disorders (CAAD)
601 North 30th Street, Suite 2850
Omaha, Nebraska 68131
402-280-4561

978-0-595-44406-9
0-595-44406-7

www.ingramcontent.com/pod-product-compliance
Lightning Source LLC
Chambersburg PA
CBHW030354290526
45785CB00004B/1740